HERBAL RECIPES

FOR

PREGNANT WOMEN

Natural Remedies for a Healthy Journey to Motherhood

Ryan Hale

Copyright © 2024 by Ryan Hale

TABLE OF CONTENTS

INTRODUCTION

WELCOME TO HERBAL RECIPES

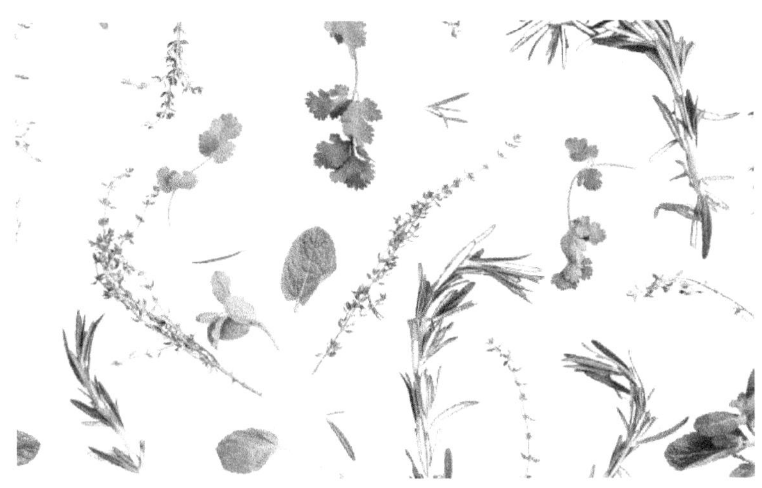

As I watched my wife, Zipporah, blossom into motherhood, I was filled with a mix of excitement and concern. Every day brought new challenges as she navigated the beautiful yet often overwhelming journey of pregnancy. From the moment we discovered we were expecting, I wanted to do everything in my power to support her and our growing baby.

In those early weeks, Zipporah experienced relentless morning sickness that left her feeling drained and discouraged. I remember the nights when she would lie in bed, clutching her stomach, wishing for relief. It broke my heart to see her struggle, and I knew I had to find a way to help.

That's when I turned to nature. I began researching herbal remedies that had been used for centuries to ease pregnancy discomforts. With each discovery, I felt a spark of hope. I started experimenting in our kitchen, crafting soothing teas infused with ginger and peppermint to combat her nausea. The first time Zipporah took a sip, her eyes lit up with surprise as she felt the gentle relief wash over her.

As the months went by, we explored the world of herbal medicine together. We learned about nourishing broths rich in vitamins and minerals that would support both her health and our baby's development. We created calming herbal teas that helped her unwind after long days filled with anticipation and preparation.

Through this journey, I realized that herbal remedies were not just about alleviating discomfort; they were about nurturing our bond as a couple and embracing the beauty of natural healing. Each recipe we crafted became a symbol of love—a testament to our commitment to a healthy pregnancy.

The Importance of Herbal Remedies During Pregnancy

This experience inspired me to compile our findings into "Herbal Recipes for Pregnant women." This book is more than just a collection of recipes; it is a heartfelt guide designed to empower expectant mothers like Zipporah to embrace the wisdom of nature during one of life's most transformative journeys.

In these pages, you will find safe and effective herbal remedies tailored for every stage of pregnancy—recipes that have brought comfort and joy into our home. Whether you are seeking relief from morning sickness, looking for ways to boost your energy, or simply wanting to nourish your body with nature's best, this book is here for you.

Join us on this journey toward holistic wellness and discover how simple herbal recipes can enhance your pregnancy experience. Let "Herbal Recipes for Pregnant women" be your trusted companion as you navigate this incredible chapter in your life—just as it was for us.

The use of herbal remedies during pregnancy has gained significant attention as expectant mothers seek natural alternatives to manage common discomforts and promote overall wellbeing. While the journey of pregnancy is filled with joy and anticipation, it can also present various physical and emotional challenges. As such, many women turn to herbal solutions to alleviate symptoms such as nausea, fatigue, anxiety, and digestive issues.

Benefits of Herbal Remedies

1. Natural Relief: Herbal remedies often provide a gentler approach to managing pregnancy related ailments compared to conventional medications. For instance, ginger is widely recognized for its effectiveness in reducing nausea and vomiting, making it a popular choice for morning sickness. Similarly, peppermint can help ease digestive discomfort and nausea, offering a soothing option for many women.

2. Nutritional Support: Many herbs are rich in vitamins and minerals that can support both maternal health and fetal development. For example, red raspberry leaf is known to tone the uterus and may help prepare the body for labor, while chamomile can promote relaxation and improve sleep quality.

3. Holistic Approach: Herbal remedies align with a holistic approach to health, addressing not only physical symptoms but also emotional wellbeing. The calming properties of certain herbs can help reduce stress and anxiety during pregnancy, fostering a sense of tranquility for both mother and baby.

4. Cultural Traditions: The use of herbal medicine is deeply rooted in various cultural practices around the world. Many women draw on traditional knowledge passed down through generations,

finding comfort in familiar remedies that have been used safely by their ancestors.

Safety Considerations

While herbal remedies can offer numerous benefits, it is essential to approach their use with caution during pregnancy. Not all herbs are safe for expectant mothers; some can have adverse effects on maternal and fetal health. Therefore, it is crucial for pregnant women to consult healthcare providers before incorporating any herbal remedies into their routine.

Research indicates that the prevalence of herbal medicine use among pregnant women varies widely across different regions and cultures. Studies show that many women utilize herbs for common pregnancy related symptoms, yet there remains a need for greater awareness regarding which herbs are safe and effective.

Herbal remedies can play a valuable role in supporting pregnant women through their unique challenges. By offering natural relief from common discomforts and promoting overall wellness, these remedies empower expectant mothers to embrace their pregnancies with confidence. However, safety must always be a priority; informed decisions based on reliable guidance are essential for ensuring both maternal and fetal health. As interest in holistic approaches continues to grow, "Herbal Recipes for Pregnant women" aims to provide expectant mothers with the knowledge they need to navigate this journey safely and effectively.

How to Use This Book

This book is designed to be a practical and accessible resource for expectant mothers seeking natural remedies to support their health and wellbeing during pregnancy. Here's how to make the most of the information and recipes contained within these pages:

1. Familiarize Yourself with the Structure

The book is organized into clear chapters, each focusing on different aspects of herbal remedies during pregnancy. Start by browsing the Table of Contents to identify sections that resonate with your current needs or interests.

2. Understand Herbal Safety

Before diving into the recipes, take time to read the sections on herbal safety and precautions. Not all herbs are suitable for every stage of pregnancy, so understanding which herbs are safe and which should be avoided is crucial for your health and the health of your baby.

3. Explore Herbal Profiles

Each chapter includes profiles of key herbs, detailing their benefits, nutritional properties, and safe usage guidelines. Familiarize yourself with these profiles to better understand how each herb can support your pregnancy journey.

4. Follow Recipes Carefully

When trying out the herbal recipes, follow the instructions closely to ensure proper preparation and dosage. Each recipe includes a list of ingredients, step-by-step instructions, and any special notes regarding preparation methods or storage.

5. Personalize Your Experience

Feel free to adapt the recipes based on your preferences and dietary needs. If you have allergies or specific health concerns, consult with a healthcare provider before making any substitutions.

6. Take Notes

As you experiment with different recipes, consider keeping a journal to track what works best for you. Note any changes in how you feel after using particular remedies, as this can help you identify what suits your body best.

7. Consult Healthcare Professionals

While this book provides valuable information and recipes, it is essential to consult with your healthcare provider before incorporating new herbal remedies into your routine. They can offer health advice based on your individual needs.

By approaching this book as a guide rather than a strict manual, you can empower yourself with knowledge and tools that promote a healthy pregnancy experience. Embrace the wisdom of nature as you explore these herbal recipes and enjoy the journey toward motherhood.

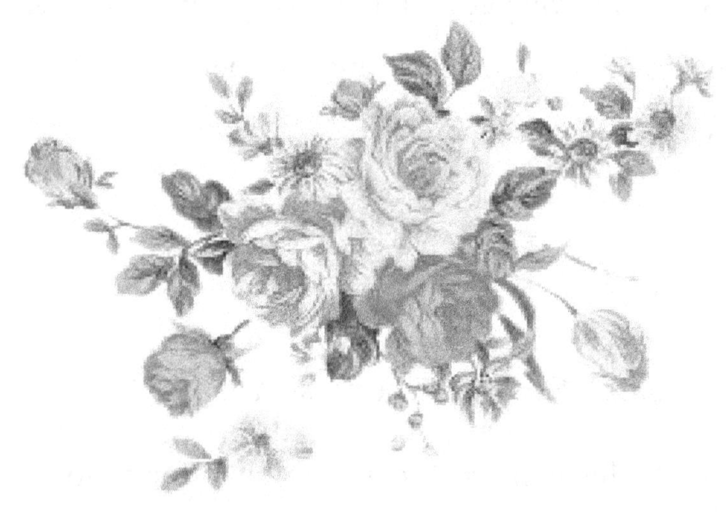

CHAPTER 1

UNDERSTANDING HERBAL MEDICINE

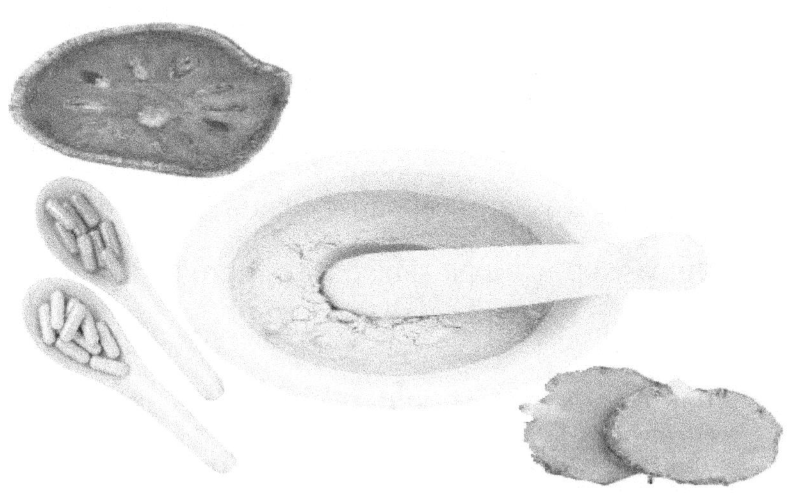

What is Herbal Medicine?

Herbal medicine, also known as botanical medicine or phytomedicine, refers to the use of plants and plant extracts for therapeutic purposes. This practice has a rich history that spans thousands of years, with roots in ancient cultures worldwide.

Today, herbal medicine is increasingly recognized for its potential benefits in promoting health and treating various conditions.

Herbal medicine encompasses a wide range of products derived from different parts of plants, including leaves, flowers, roots, seeds, and bark. These natural compounds may be used in various forms such as teas, capsules, tinctures, powders, and topical applications. The active ingredients in these herbal preparations can offer therapeutic benefits, making them a popular choice for individuals seeking natural alternatives to conventional medications.

Historical Context

The use of herbal remedies dates back to ancient civilizations, including those in China, Egypt, and India. Historical texts reveal that many cultures relied on plants for healing long before the advent of modern pharmaceuticals. For instance, Traditional Chinese Medicine (TCM) and Ayurveda are two well-established systems that utilize herbs as a core component of their therapeutic practices.

Modern Usage

In contemporary society, herbal medicine is often categorized as complementary and alternative medicine (CAM). Many people turn to herbal remedies to address various health issues, including chronic conditions such as anxiety, digestive disorders, and inflammation. According to estimates from the World Health Organization (WHO), approximately 80% of the global population relies on herbal medicines for some aspect of their health care.

Benefits of Herbal Medicine

Natural Healing: Herbal remedies are often perceived as safer alternatives to synthetic drugs. Many individuals prefer using herbs due to their natural origins and fewer side effects when compared to conventional medications.

Holistic Approach: Herbal medicine typically emphasizes a holistic approach to health, focusing on the overall wellbeing of the individual rather than merely treating specific symptoms or diseases.

Cultural Relevance: In many cultures, herbal medicine is deeply integrated into traditional healing practices. The knowledge passed down through generations continues to influence modern approaches to health care.

Herbal medicine is essential for anyone interested in exploring natural remedies, especially during pregnancy. Herbal medicine, also known as botanical or phytomedicine, involves the use of various parts of plants—such as seeds, roots, leaves, flowers, and bark—for therapeutic purposes. This practice has a rich history that dates back thousands of years, with roots in ancient cultures worldwide, including Traditional Chinese Medicine and Ayurveda.

The Significance of Herbal Medicine

Herbal medicine plays a crucial role in health care systems globally, with an estimated 80% of the world's population relying on herbal remedies for their primary health care needs. This reliance is particularly pronounced in regions where access to conventional medical treatments is limited. The growing interest in herbal medicine reflects a desire for more natural and holistic approaches to health, especially among those who seek alternatives to pharmaceutical drugs.

The Future of Herbal Medicine

The acceptance of herbal medicine is growing within mainstream healthcare as more practitioners recognize its potential benefits. Research into the efficacy and safety of various herbs continues to expand, paving the way for more informed use in clinical settings. As healthcare providers become more educated about herbal remedies, they can better guide patients in integrating these natural solutions into their overall health plans.

In summary, understanding herbal medicine is crucial for anyone interested in exploring its benefits, particularly during pregnancy. With a rich history and a growing body of research supporting its use, herbal remedies offer a promising complement to conventional medical practices. However, safety must always be a priority; informed decisions based on reliable guidance are essential for ensuring both maternal and fetal health.

Embracing the wisdom of herbal medicine can enhance the pregnancy experience, providing natural support as you embark on this remarkable journey toward motherhood.

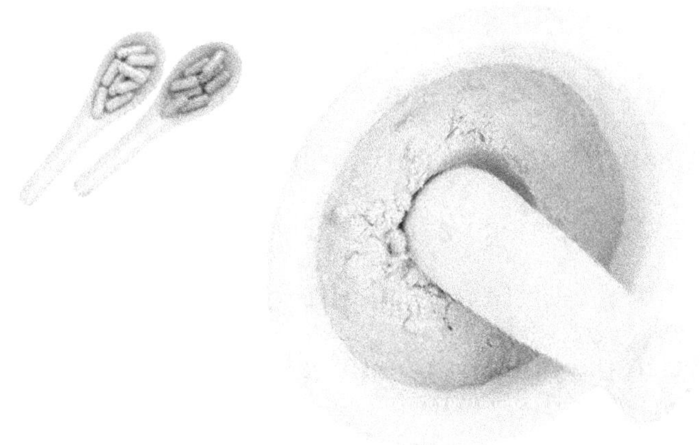

Benefits of Using Herbs During Pregnancy

Here's a powerful section on the Benefits of Using Herbs During Pregnancy, drawing from the search results and general knowledge about herbal medicine.

The use of herbal remedies during pregnancy has gained popularity as more expectant mothers seek natural alternatives to manage common discomforts and enhance their overall wellbeing. While it is essential to approach herbal medicine with caution, the potential benefits are significant and can make a positive impact on both maternal and fetal health.

1. Natural Relief from Common Ailments

Pregnancy often brings a host of physical challenges, including nausea, vomiting, fatigue, and digestive issues. Herbal remedies such as ginger and peppermint are renowned for their effectiveness in alleviating morning sickness and digestive discomfort. Studies have shown that ginger can significantly reduce nausea without adverse effects when used in appropriate doses, making it a safe option for many pregnant women.

2. Support for Emotional Wellbeing

The emotional rollercoaster of pregnancy can lead to anxiety and stress. Certain herbs, like chamomile and lemon balm, are known for their calming effects, helping to promote relaxation and improve sleep quality. By incorporating these soothing herbs into their routines, expectant mothers can find relief from stress and anxiety, fostering a more positive pregnancy experience.

3. Nutritional Benefits

Many herbs are rich in essential vitamins and minerals that support both maternal health and fetal development. For example, red raspberry leaf is often recommended for its potential benefits in toning the uterus and preparing the body for labor. Additionally, herbs like nettle provide valuable nutrients such as iron and calcium, which are crucial during pregnancy.

4. Holistic Approach to Health

Herbal medicine embodies a holistic approach that considers the whole person—body, mind, and spirit. This perspective aligns well with the needs of pregnant women seeking comprehensive care that addresses not just physical symptoms but also emotional and psychological wellbeing. By using herbs as part of a holistic health plan, women can empower themselves to take an active role in their pregnancy journey.

5. Cultural Significance and Accessibility

Herbal remedies have been used for centuries across various cultures, often passed down through generations as traditional knowledge. This cultural significance lends credibility to their use during pregnancy. Additionally, many herbal products are easily accessible and can be obtained without a prescription, making them appealing options for expectant mothers seeking immediate relief.

6. Potential for Fewer Side Effects

Many pregnant women prefer herbal remedies over pharmaceutical options due to the perception that they are safer for both mother and baby. While it is crucial to remember that "natural" does not always mean "safe," many herbs have been used traditionally with fewer reported side effects compared to conventional medications. However, it is still essential to consult healthcare providers before using any herbal products.

7. Empowerment Through Knowledge

Using herbs during pregnancy encourages women to educate themselves about natural health practices. This empowerment fosters a sense of control over one's health choices during a time when many feel vulnerable due to physical changes and uncertainties about childbirth. Understanding how different herbs work allows expectant mothers to make informed decisions tailored to their specific needs.

8. Enhanced Connection with Nature

Incorporating herbal remedies into daily routines can deepen an expectant mother's connection with nature. This relationship not only promotes emotional wellbeing but also instills a sense of respect for the natural world and its healing properties. Engaging with nature through gardening or simply enjoying herbal teas made from fresh ingredients can be a therapeutic practice in itself.

In summary, the benefits of using herbs during pregnancy are multifaceted, offering natural relief from common ailments while supporting emotional wellbeing and nutritional health. As interest in holistic approaches continues to grow, herbal remedies present an appealing option for expectant mothers looking to enhance their pregnancy experience. However, safety should always be a priority; informed decisions based on reliable guidance are essential for ensuring both maternal and fetal health.

Safety Considerations and Precautions

While herbal remedies can offer numerous benefits during pregnancy, it is crucial to approach their use with caution. The perception that herbal products are inherently safe can be misleading, as many herbs contain active compounds that may affect both maternal and fetal health. Understanding the safety considerations associated with herbal medicine is essential for expectant mothers.

Potential Risks of Herbal Use

Herbal medicines can carry risks, including:

Teratogenicity: Some herbs may cause birth defects or developmental issues in the fetus. For instance, certain herbs known as emmenagogues, like blue cohosh and black cohosh, can stimulate uterine contractions and potentially lead to complications such as miscarriage or premature labor.

Hormonal Effects: Many herbs can influence hormonal levels, which may impact fetal development or maternal health. For example, herbs like fenugreek and licorice have been associated with hormonal changes that could pose risks during pregnancy.

Increased Bleeding Risk: Some herbal remedies may increase the risk of bleeding, particularly during labor. Herbs such as shepherd's purse are known for their blood clotting properties but can also pose risks if not used correctly.

Lack of Regulation and Research

Herbal products are often sold as dietary supplements and are not subject to the same rigorous testing and regulation as pharmaceutical drugs. This lack of oversight raises concerns about:

Contamination: Herbal products may be contaminated with heavy metals, pesticides, or other harmful substances due to poor manufacturing practices.

Variable Potency: The concentration of active ingredients in herbal products can vary widely between brands and batches, leading to inconsistent effects and potential overdosing or under dosing.

Limited Research: There is a significant lack of randomized controlled trials (RCTs) specifically evaluating the safety and efficacy of many commonly used herbs during pregnancy. Most available studies focus on a limited number of herbs, such as ginger and raspberry leaf, leaving many other herbal remedies unstudied.

Herb Drug Interactions

Expectant mothers often take other medications or supplements during pregnancy. Herbal remedies can interact with these substances, leading to:

Altered Drug Efficacy: Some herbs may enhance or inhibit the effects of prescribed medications, which could complicate treatment plans for conditions like hypertension or diabetes.

Unexpected Side Effects: The combination of herbal products with conventional medications may result in adverse reactions that could affect both mother and baby.

Consultation with Healthcare Providers

Given the potential risks associated with herbal use during pregnancy, it is vital for expectant mothers to:

Communicate Openly: Always inform healthcare providers about any herbal remedies being used. This transparency allows for better monitoring and management of potential interactions or side effects.

Seek Professional Guidance: Consult healthcare professionals who are knowledgeable about herbal medicine before starting any new herbal regimen. They can provide evidence-based recommendations tailored to individual health needs.

Educating Yourself

Expectant mothers should take the initiative to educate themselves about:

Safe Herbs: Familiarize yourself with herbs that are considered safe during pregnancy, such as ginger for nausea or peppermint for digestive issues.

Dosage Guidelines: Understand appropriate dosages for safe use, as some herbs may be safe in small amounts but harmful in larger quantities.

Recognizing Side Effects: Be aware of potential side effects associated with specific herbs and monitor any changes in health closely.

In conclusion, while herbal remedies can provide valuable support during pregnancy, it is essential to prioritize safety through informed decision making. By understanding the potential risks associated with herbal use, consulting healthcare providers, and educating themselves about safe practices, expectant mothers can navigate their options confidently. Embracing a cautious approach will help ensure the wellbeing of both mother and baby throughout this remarkable journey.

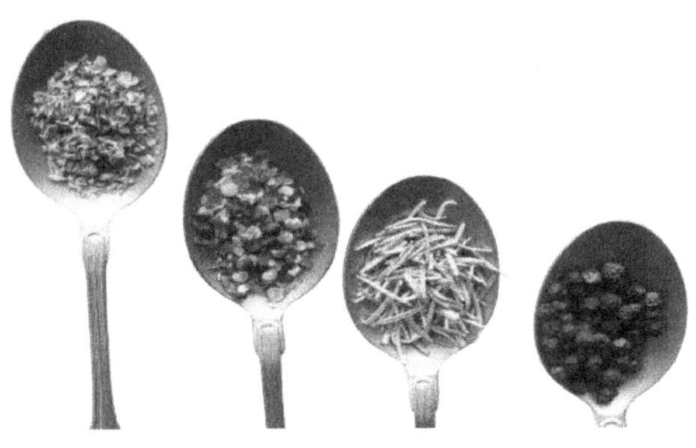

CHAPTER 2

ESSENTIAL HERBS FOR PREGNANCY

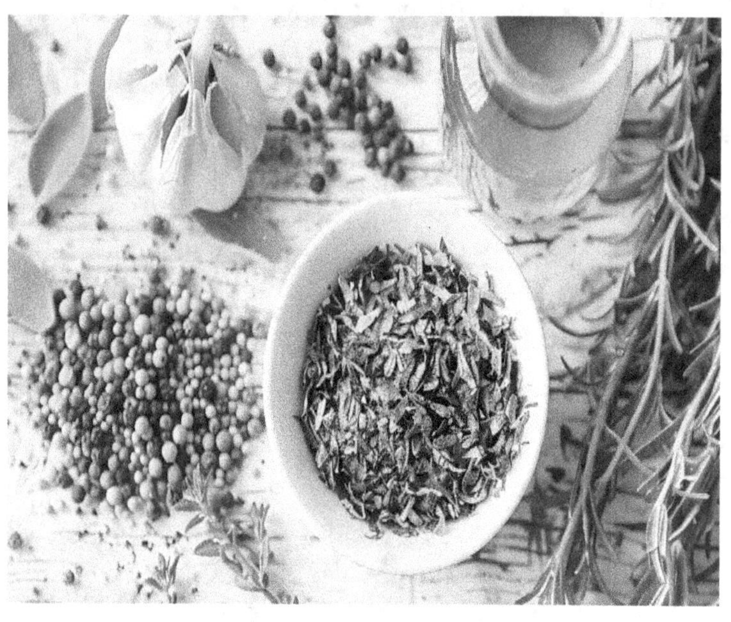

The journey of pregnancy is a transformative experience that often comes with various physical and emotional challenges. Many expectant mothers turn to herbal remedies as a natural means of alleviating common discomforts and supporting their overall health. Essential herbs such as ginger, peppermint, and red raspberry leaf have been used for centuries for their therapeutic properties. These herbs can provide relief from nausea, promote relaxation, and even support uterine health. However, it is crucial for pregnant women to approach herbal use with caution, ensuring they consult healthcare providers to understand which herbs are safe and beneficial during this unique time. By incorporating the right herbal remedies, expectant mothers can enhance their wellbeing and embrace the beauty of their pregnancy journey.

Overview of Key Herbs

Herbal remedies have been utilized for centuries to support health and alleviate common discomforts during pregnancy. While many herbs are considered safe, it is crucial for expectant mothers to consult healthcare providers before incorporating them into their routines. Below is an overview of some key herbs that are frequently used during pregnancy.

1. Red Raspberry Leaf (Rubus idaeus)
2. Ginger (Zingiber officinale)
3. Peppermint (Mentha piperita)
4. Chamomile (Matricaria chamomilla)
5. Thyme (Thymus vulgaris)
6. Dandelion (Taraxacum officinale)
7. Lemon Balm (Melissa officinalis)
8. Oat Straw (Avena sativa)
9. Fenugreek (Trigonella foenumgraecum)
10. Echinacea (Echinacea purpurea)
11. Linden (Tilia spp.)
12. Sage (Salvia officinalis)
13. Ashwagandha (Withania somnifera)
14. Shatavari (Asparagus racemosus)
15. Nettle (Urtica dioica)
16. Hibiscus (Hibiscus sabdariffa)
17. Fennel (Foeniculum vulgare)

18. Milk Thistle (Silybum marianum)

19. Burdock Root (Arctium lappa)

20. Alfalfa (Medicago sativa)

21. Moringa (Moringa oleifera)

22. Calendula (Calendula officinalis)

23. Catnip (Nepeta cataria)

24. Valerian Root (Valeriana officinalis)

25. Passionflower (Passiflora incarnata)

26. Cinnamon (Cinnamomum verum)

27. Clary Sage (Salvia sclarea)

28. Ginseng (Panax ginseng or Panax quinquefolius)

29. Holy Basil (Ocimum sanctum or Ocimum tenuiflorum)

30. Rosemary (Rosmarinus officinalis)

This list provides a diverse range of herbs that may be beneficial during pregnancy, but it is essential for expectant mothers to consult healthcare providers before using any herbal remedies to ensure safety and appropriate individual health needs.

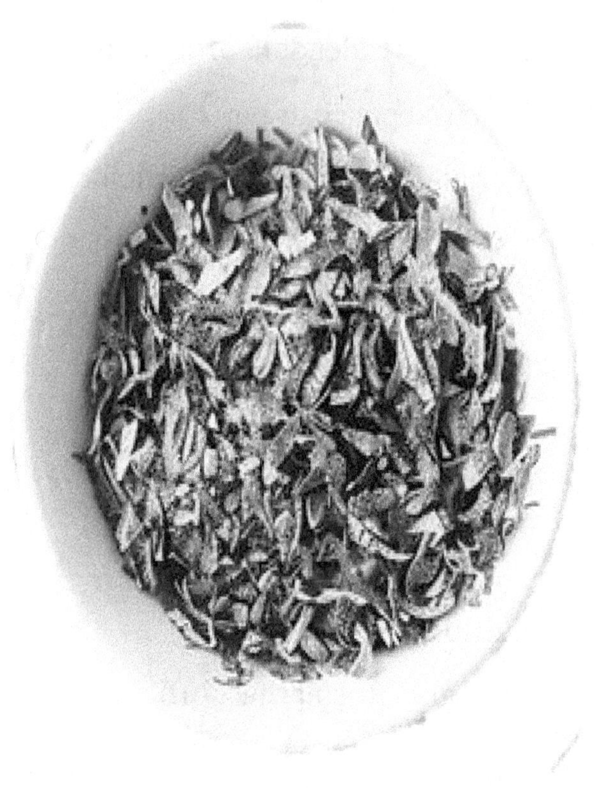

Nutritional Benefits of Each Herb

1.Red Raspberry Leaf (Rubus idaeus)

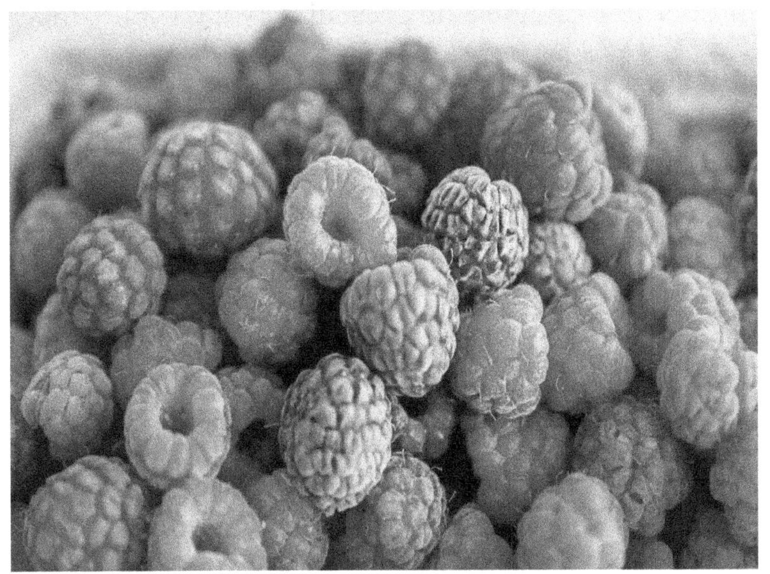

Vitamins: Rich in vitamins C, E, A, and B, which are essential for immune function and overall health.

Minerals: Contains calcium, iron, potassium, and magnesium. Calcium provide supportive bone health, while iron is vital for red blood cell production.

Plant Compounds: High in tannins and flavonoids that offer antioxidant and antiinflammatory properties. Ellagic acid present may have anticancer effects.

Benefits: Traditionally used to tone the uterus and may help with labor efficiency. It also supports digestive health and provides antioxidant protection.

2. Ginger (Zingiber officinale)

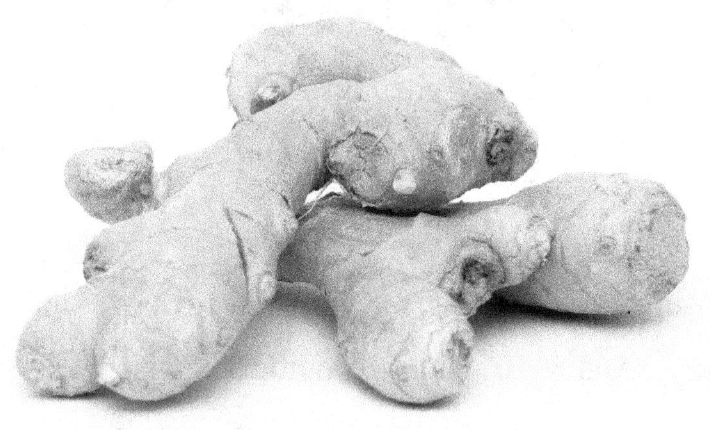

Vitamins: Contains small amounts of vitamin B6, which is important for brain development.

Minerals: Provides potassium and magnesium, aiding in electrolyte balance.

Bioactive Compounds: Rich in gingerol and other antioxidants with antiinflammatory effects.

Benefits: Effective in reducing nausea and vomiting during pregnancy.

3.Peppermint (Mentha piperita)

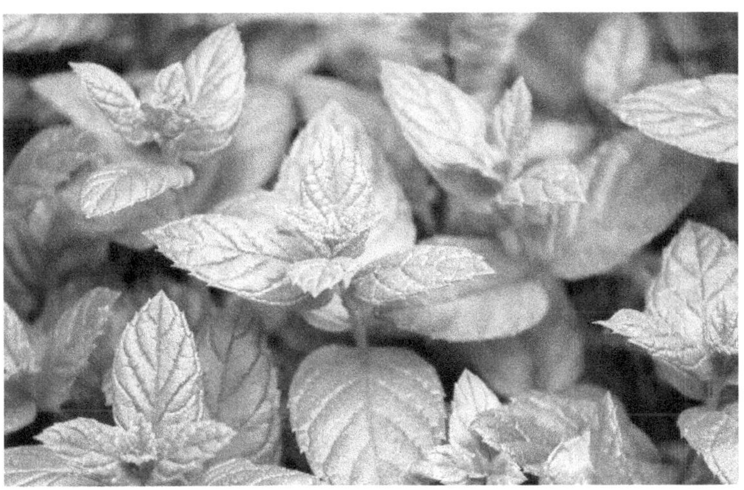

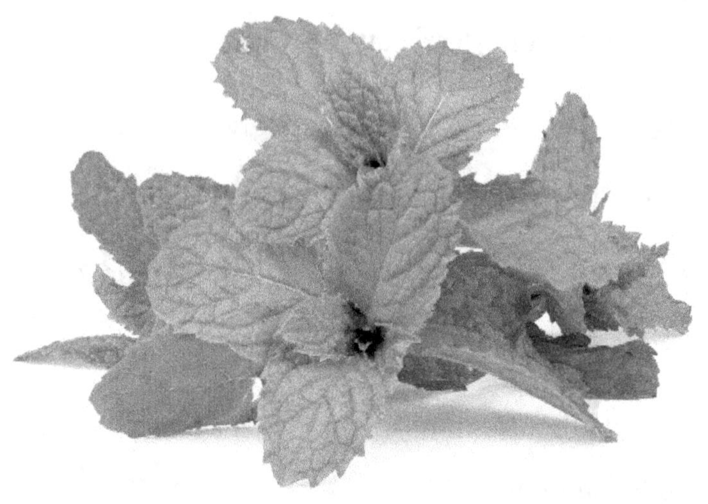

Vitamins: Contains small amounts of vitamins A and C.

Minerals: Provides potassium and calcium.

Essential Oils: Rich in menthol, which soothes the digestive system.

Benefits: Known for relieving nausea and indigestion; promotes relaxation.

4.Chamomile (Matricaria chamomilla)

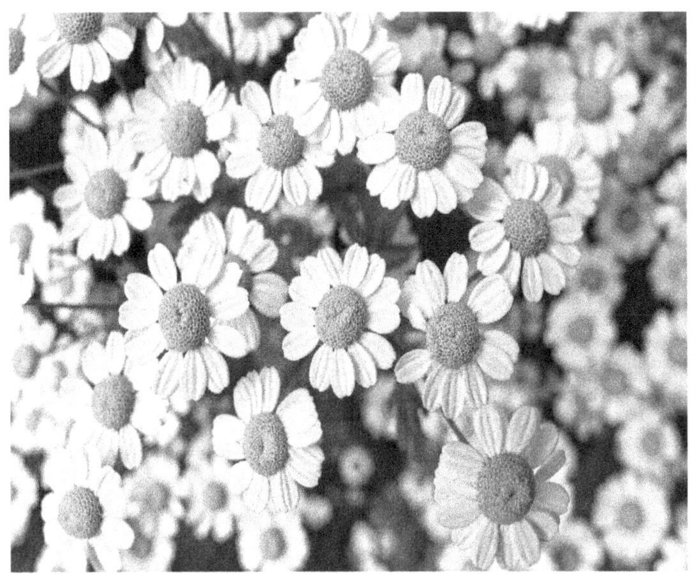

Vitamins & Minerals: Contains calcium, potassium, and magnesium.

Antioxidants: Rich in flavonoids that provide antiinflammatory benefits.

Benefits: Helps promote relaxation and improve sleep quality; may aid in digestion.

5.Cranberry (Vaccinium macrocarpon)

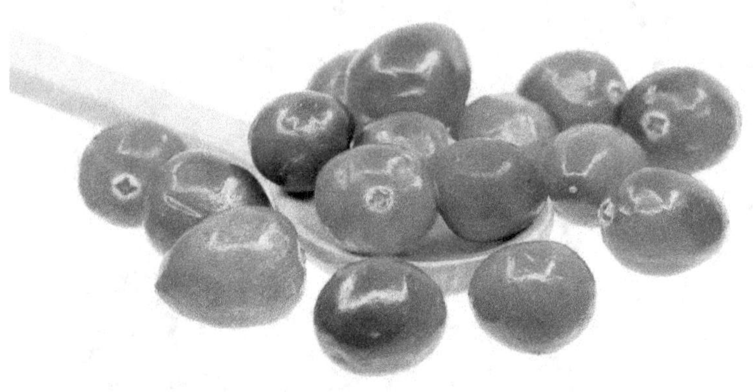

Vitamins: High in vitamin C, supporting immune health.

Antioxidants: Contains anthocyanins, flavonols, and flavan3ols that prevent bacterial infections, especially urinary tract infections (UTIs).

Fiber: A good source of dietary fiber aiding digestion.

Benefits: Commonly used to prevent UTIs during pregnancy.

6.Slippery Elm (Ulmus rubra)

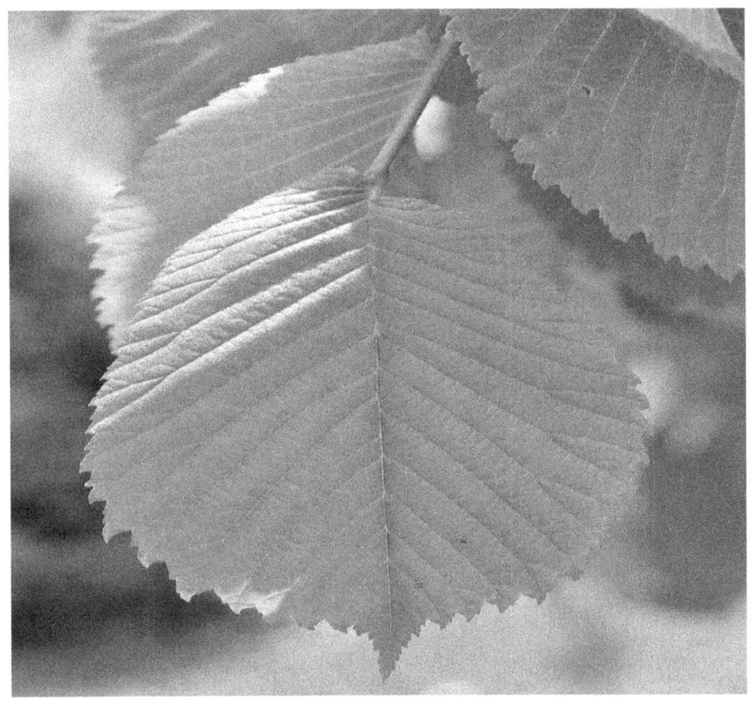

Mucilage Content: Rich in mucilage that soothes the digestive tract.

Vitamins & Minerals: Provides small amounts of calcium, potassium, and magnesium.

Benefits: Known for alleviating heartburn and gastrointestinal discomfort.

7.Thyme (Thymus vulgaris)

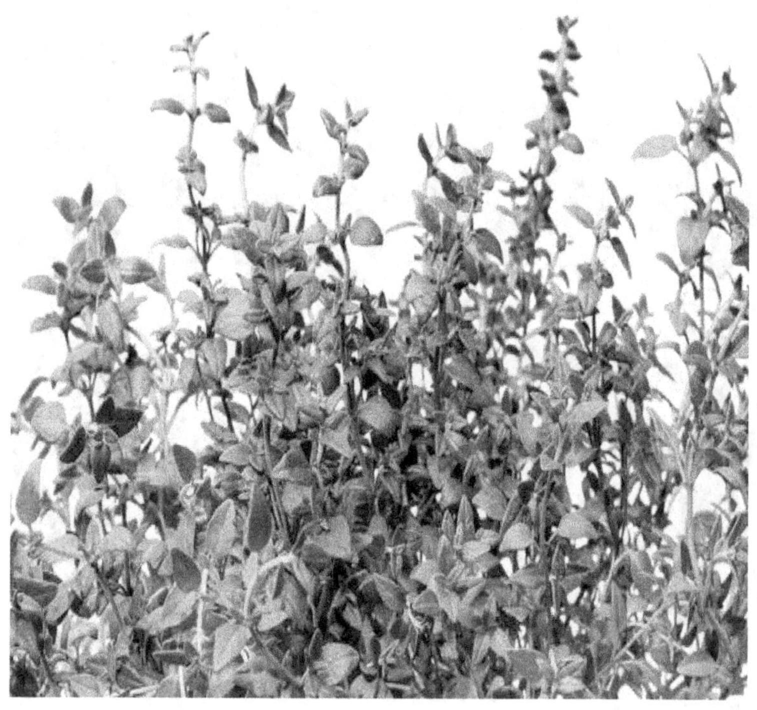

Vitamins & Minerals: Contains vitamin C and several essential minerals.

Antioxidants: Rich in flavonoids with antimicrobial properties.

Benefits: Supports respiratory health; may help alleviate coughs.

8. Dandelion (Taraxacum officinale)

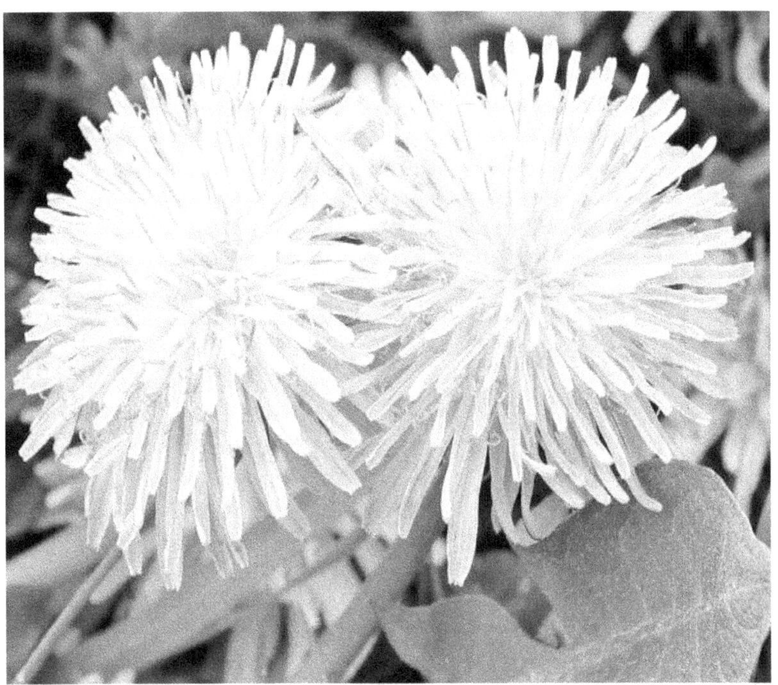

Vitamins & Minerals: High in vitamins A, C, K, and several B vitamins; rich in potassium and calcium.

Benefits: Supports liver function and aids digestion; may help reduce water retention.

9. Lemon Balm (Melissa officinalis)

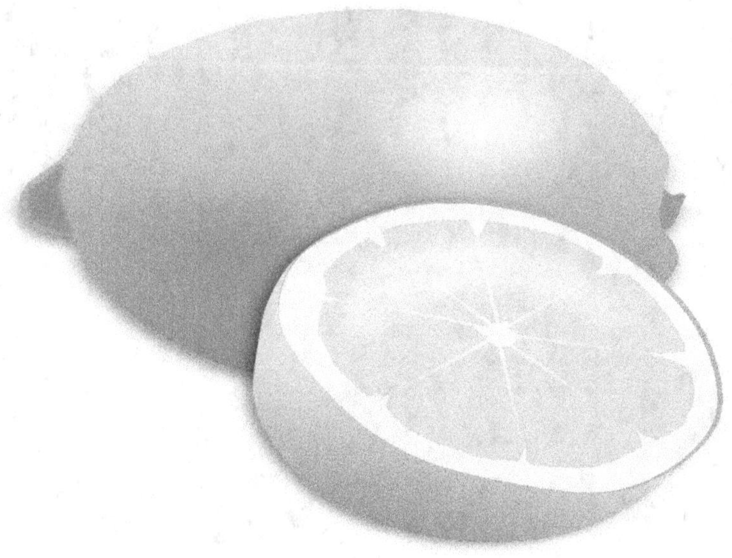

Vitamins & Minerals: Contains small amounts of vitamin C and several minerals.

Benefits: Known for its calming effects; helps reduce anxiety and promote relaxation.

10.Oat Straw (Avena sativa)

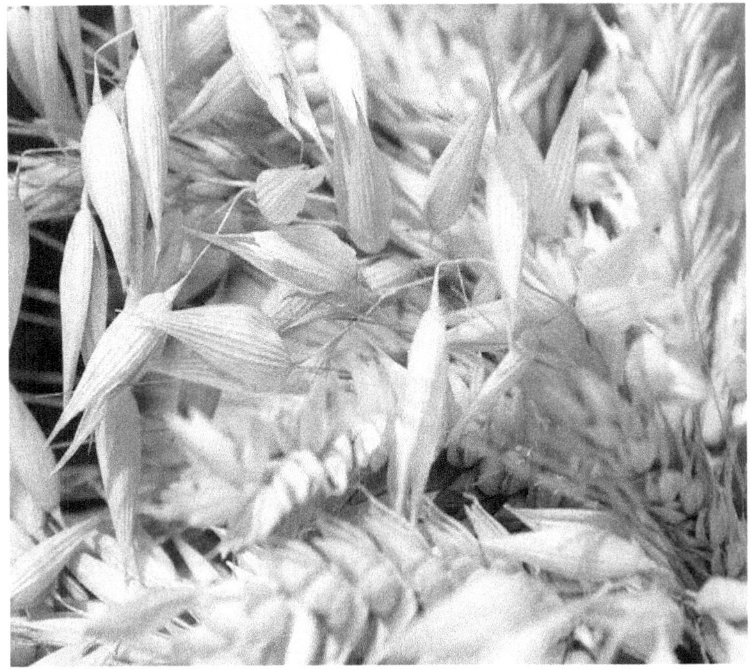

Vitamins & Minerals: Rich in calcium, magnesium, iron, and silica.

Benefits: Promotes relaxation; supports healthy skin during pregnancy.

11.Fenugreek (Trigonella foenumgraecum)

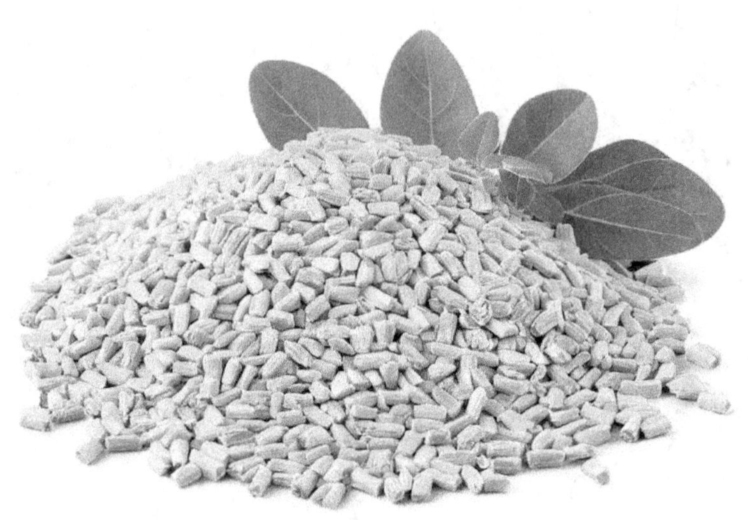

Vitamins & Minerals: Contains vitamins A, B6, C, iron, calcium, magnesium, phosphorus, potassium, and zinc.

Benefits: Traditionally used to enhance milk production in breastfeeding mothers; may help regulate blood sugar levels.

12. Echinacea (Echinacea purpurea)

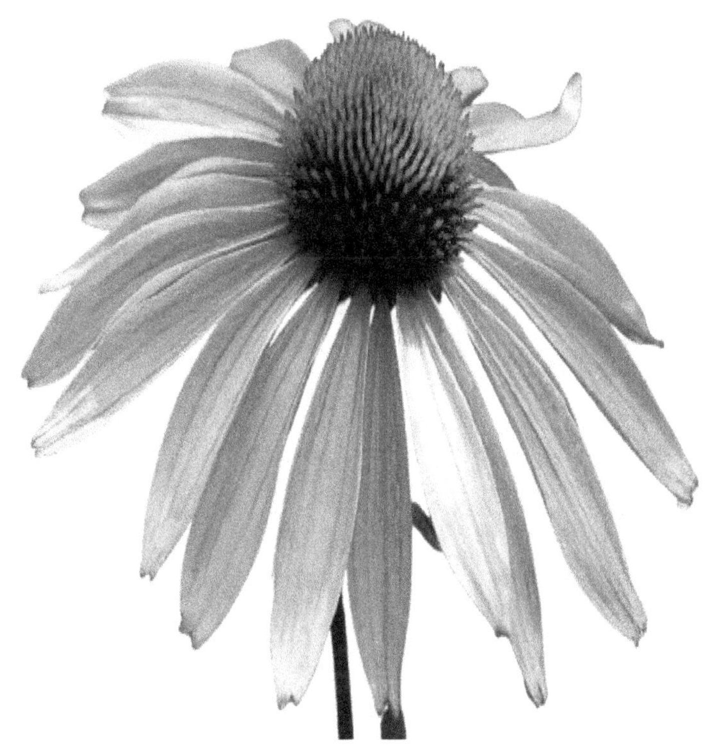

Vitamins & Minerals: Contains vitamin C and several antioxidants.

Benefits: Boosts the immune system; may help prevent colds during pregnancy.

13. Linden (Tilia spp.)

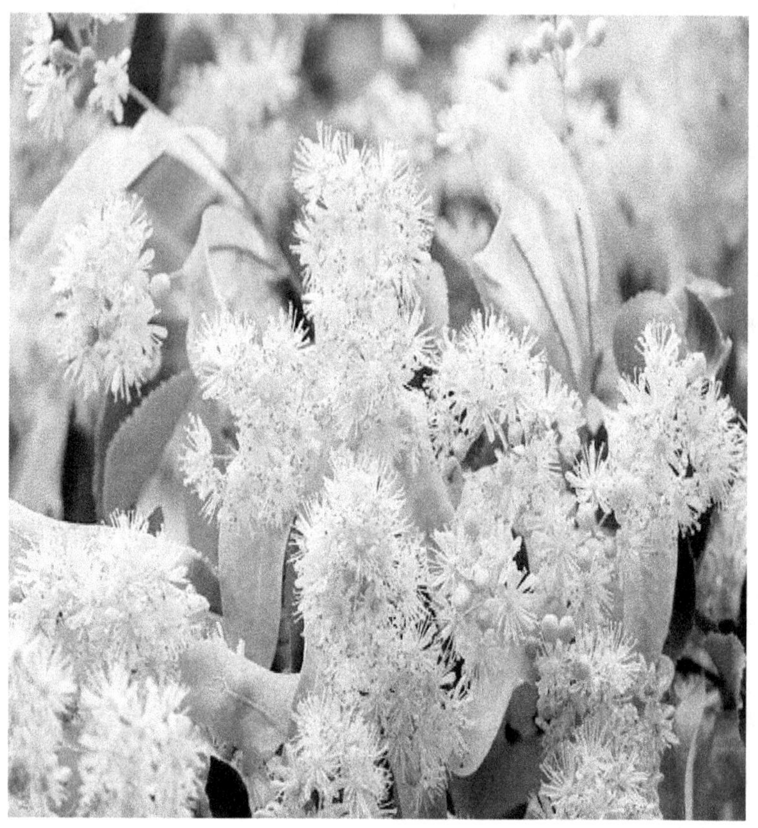

Vitamins & Minerals: Contains vitamin C and antioxidants.

Benefits: Known for its calming effects; helps relieve anxiety and promote sleep.

14.Sage (Salvia officinalis)

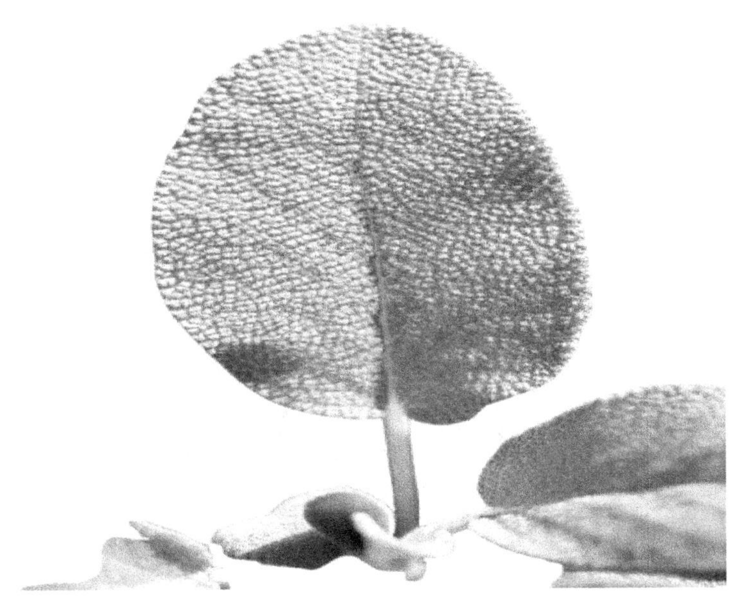

Nutrients: Contains vitamins A, C, K, calcium, magnesium, iron, and potassium.

Benefits: Antioxidant properties; may support digestive health but should be used cautiously during pregnancy due to potential uterine stimulation.

15.Ashwagandha (Withania somnifera)

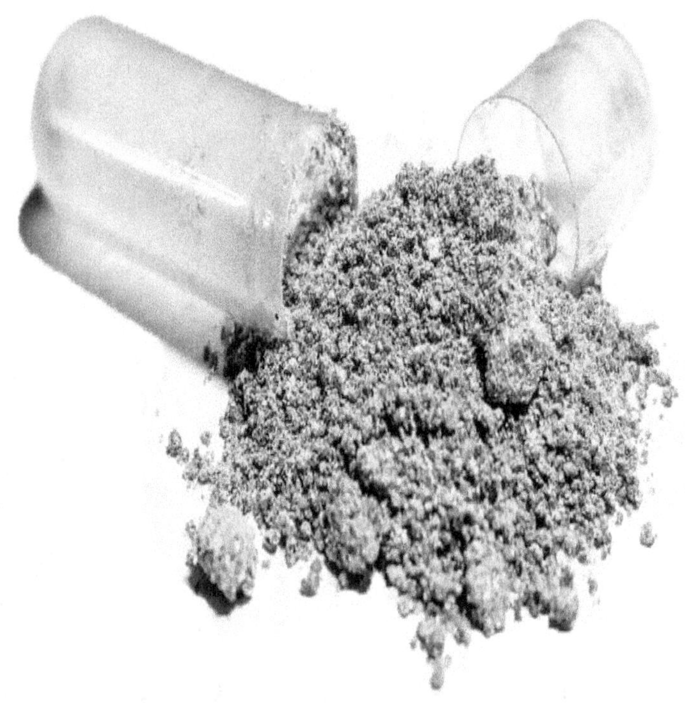

Nutrients: Contains iron, calcium, amino acids, fatty acids, alkaloids, and flavonoids.

Benefits: Adaptogenic herb that helps reduce stress; should be used under medical supervision during pregnancy.

16.Shatavari (Asparagus racemosus)

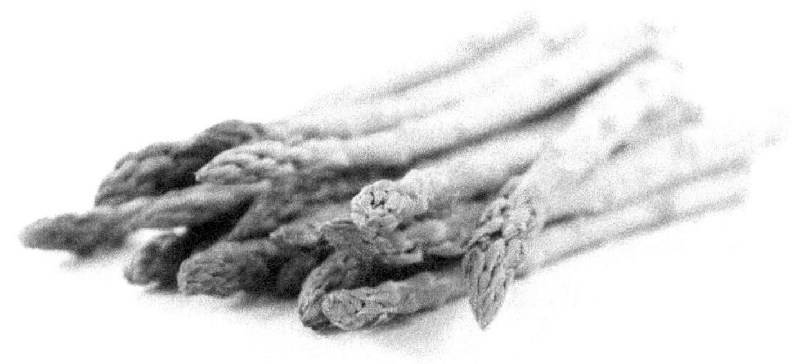

Vitamins & Minerals: Rich in vitamins A, C, and E, as well as several B vitamins. It also contains minerals like calcium, magnesium, and potassium.

Benefits: Known for its adaptogenic properties, Shatavari helps balance hormones and supports female reproductive health. It may enhance fertility and is traditionally used to improve lactation in breastfeeding mothers. Additionally, it has antioxidant properties that support immune function.

17.Nettle (Urtica dioica)

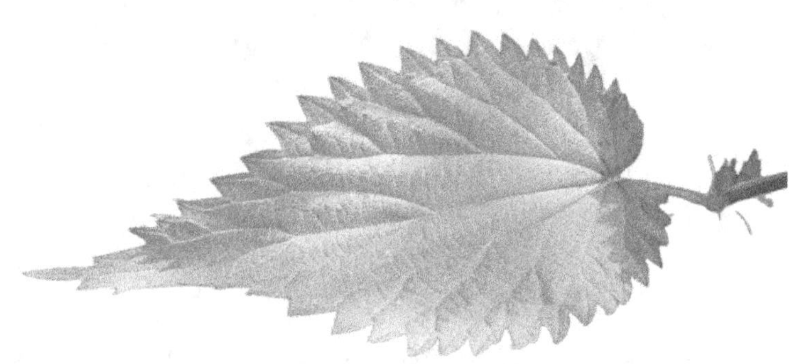

Vitamins & Minerals: Nettle is a nutrient powerhouse, providing vitamins A, C, K, and several B vitamins. It is also high in iron, calcium, magnesium, and potassium.

Benefits: Nettle is known for its ability to alleviate fatigue due to its high iron content. It may help reduce inflammation and support urinary tract health. Additionally, it can aid in digestion and provide essential nutrients that support overall health during pregnancy.

18. **Hibiscus (Hibiscus sabdariffa)**

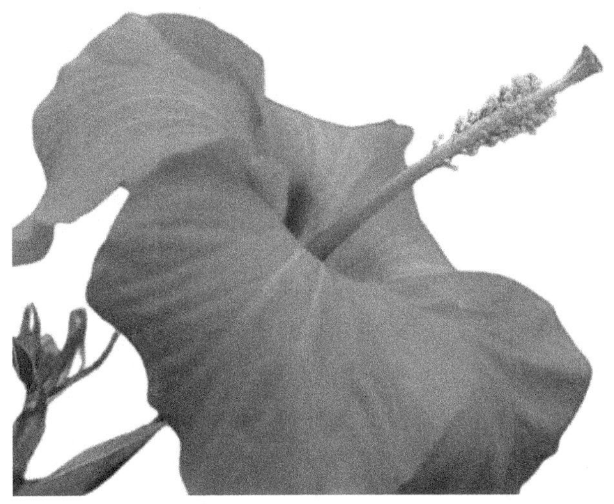

Vitamins & Minerals: Hibiscus is rich in vitamin C and antioxidants such as anthocyanins.

Benefits: Known for its potential to lower blood pressure and improve heart health, hibiscus tea can also aid digestion and provide hydration. However, it should be consumed in moderation during pregnancy due to its potential effects on blood pressure.

19.Fennel (Foeniculum vulgare)

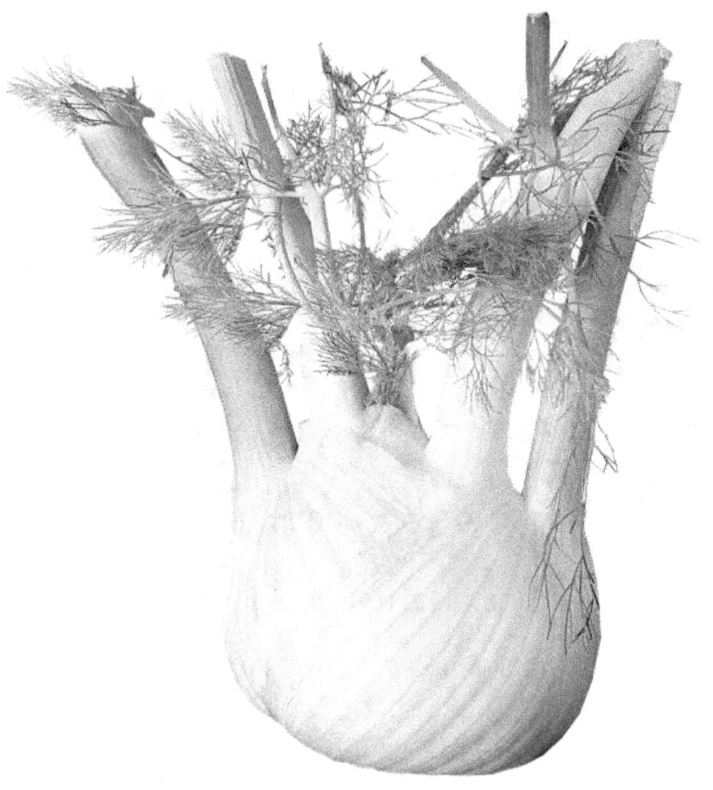

Vitamins & Minerals: Fennel is a good source of vitamins C and A, as well as minerals like potassium and calcium.

Benefits: Fennel seeds are often used to relieve digestive issues and reduce bloating. They may also help alleviate menstrual discomfort and promote milk production in breastfeeding mothers.

20.Milk Thistle (Silybum marianum)

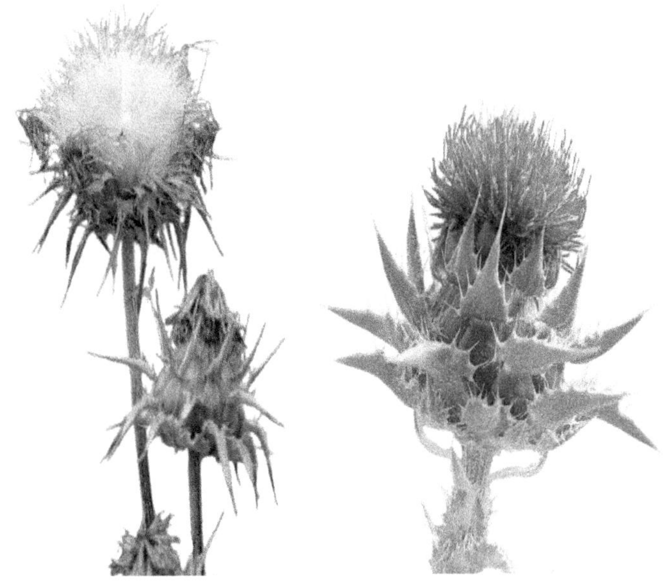

Vitamins & Minerals: Milk thistle contains silymarin, which has antioxidant properties.

Benefits: Traditionally used to support liver health, milk thistle may help detoxify the body. However, pregnant women should consult healthcare providers before use due to limited research on safety during pregnancy.

21.**Burdock Root (Arctium lappa)**

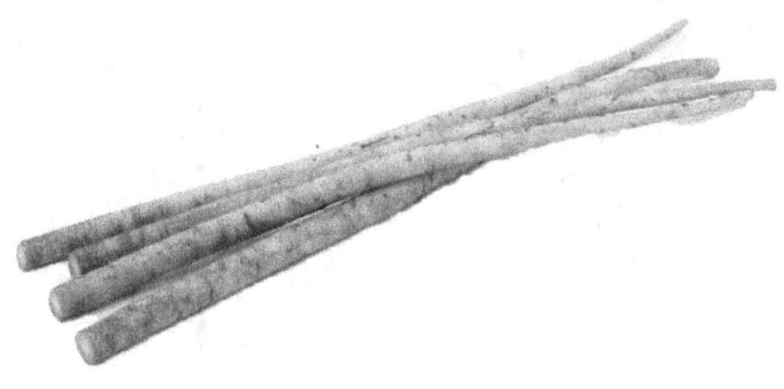

Vitamins & Minerals: Burdock root is rich in vitamins A, C, E, and several B vitamins. It also contains minerals like iron, calcium, magnesium, and potassium.

Benefits: Known for its detoxifying properties, burdock root may help purify the blood and support liver function. It has antiinflammatory properties that can benefit skin health during pregnancy.

22.Alfalfa (Medicago sativa)

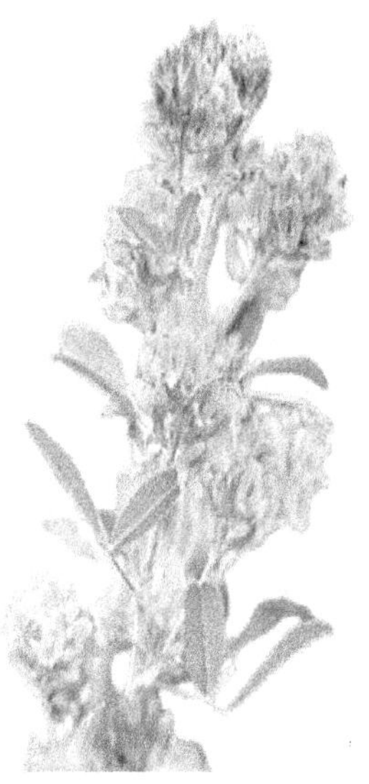

Vitamins & Minerals: Alfalfa is high in vitamins A, C, E, K, and several B vitamins. It also provides calcium, iron, magnesium, phosphorus, and potassium.

Benefits: Alfalfa is known for its ability to support overall health due to its nutrient density. It may help with digestion and provide essential nutrients that are beneficial during pregnancy.

23.**Moringa (Moringa oleifera)**

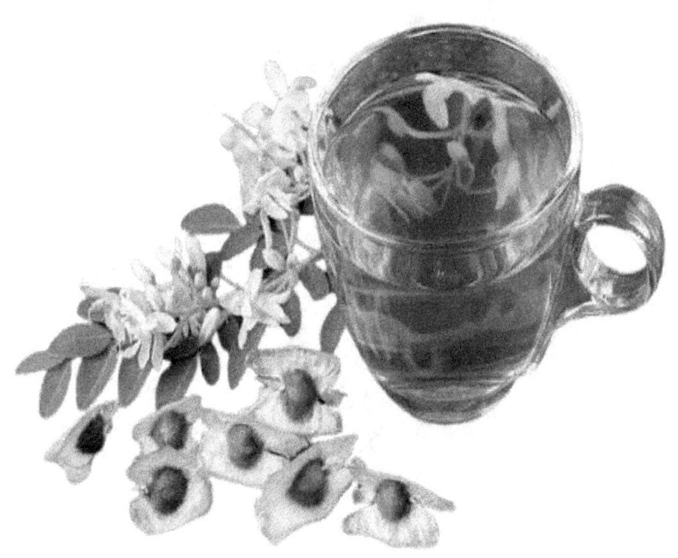

Vitamins & Minerals: Moringa leaves are exceptionally nutrient dense, containing vitamins A, C, K, and several B vitamins along with calcium, iron, magnesium, and potassium.

Benefits: Moringa is known for its antiinflammatory properties and may help boost energy levels while supporting immune function. Its high nutrient content makes it a valuable addition to a pregnant woman's diet.

24.Calendula (Calendula officinalis)

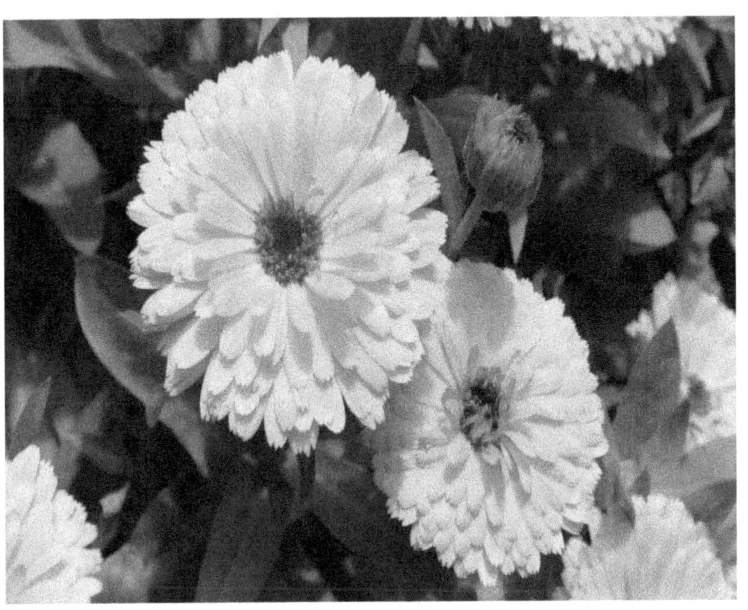

Vitamins & Minerals: Calendula contains antioxidants such as flavonoids and carotenoids.

Benefits: Often used topically for skin irritations or rashes during pregnancy; calendula may also promote healing and reduce inflammation.

25.Catnip (Nepeta cataria)

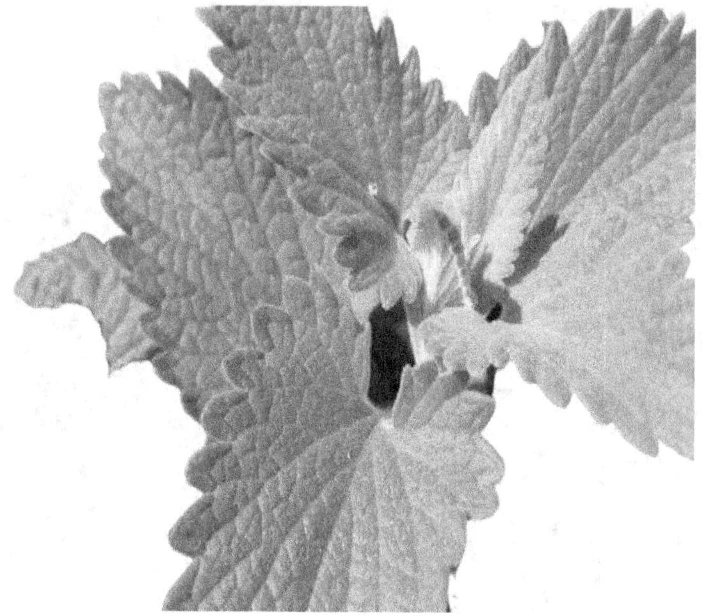

Vitamins & Minerals: Contains small amounts of vitamins A and C along with several minerals.

Benefits: Catnip is known for its calming effects; it can help relieve stress and promote relaxation during pregnancy.

26. Valerian Root (Valeriana officinalis)

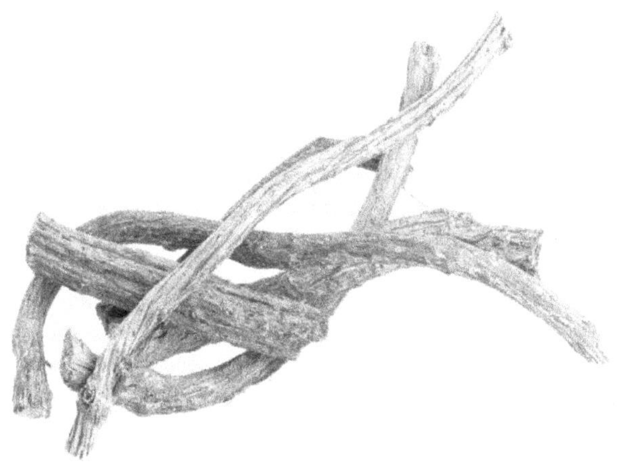

Vitamins & Minerals: Contains various phytochemicals but limited vitamin content.

Benefits: Valerian root is commonly used to promote sleep and reduce anxiety; however, pregnant women should use it cautiously under medical supervision due to limited research on safety during pregnancy.

27.Passionflower (Passiflora incarnata)

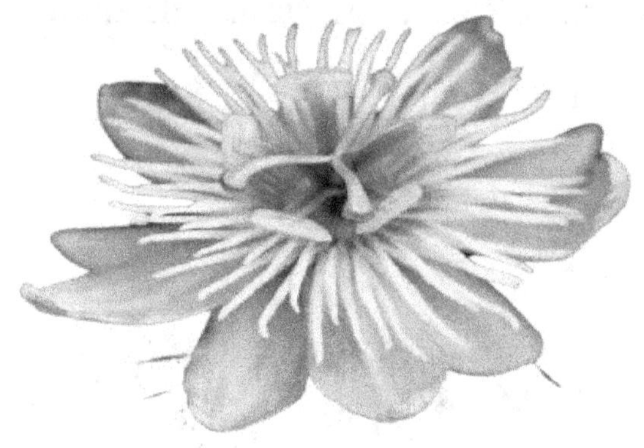

Vitamins & Minerals: Contains small amounts of various vitamins but is primarily valued for its calming compounds.

Benefits: Passionflower is known for its anxiety reducing effects; it may help promote relaxation and improve sleep quality during pregnancy.

28.Cinnamon (Cinnamomum verum)

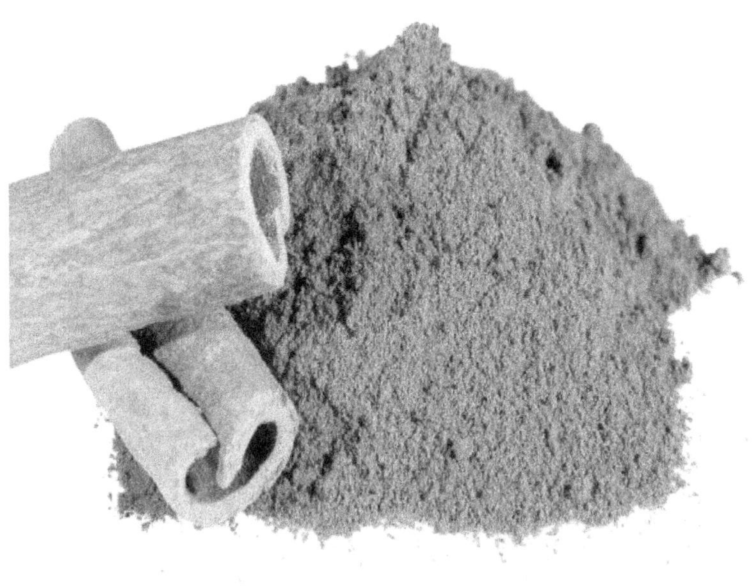

Vitamins & Minerals: Contains small amounts of calcium and manganese.

Benefits: Cinnamon has antioxidant properties that can help regulate blood sugar levels; however, it should be consumed in moderation during pregnancy.

29.Clary Sage (Salvia sclarea)

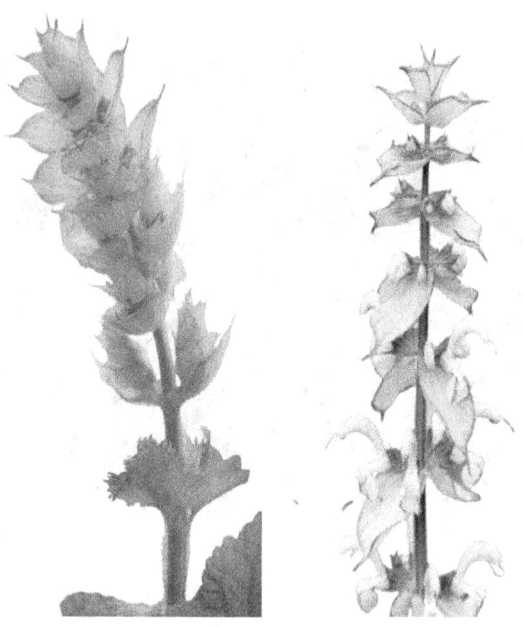

Vitamins & Minerals: Contains antioxidants but limited vitamin content.

Benefits: Clary sage is known for its potential hormonal balancing effects; however, it should be used cautiously during pregnancy due to its uterine stimulating properties.

30.Ginseng (Panax ginseng or Panax quinquefolius)

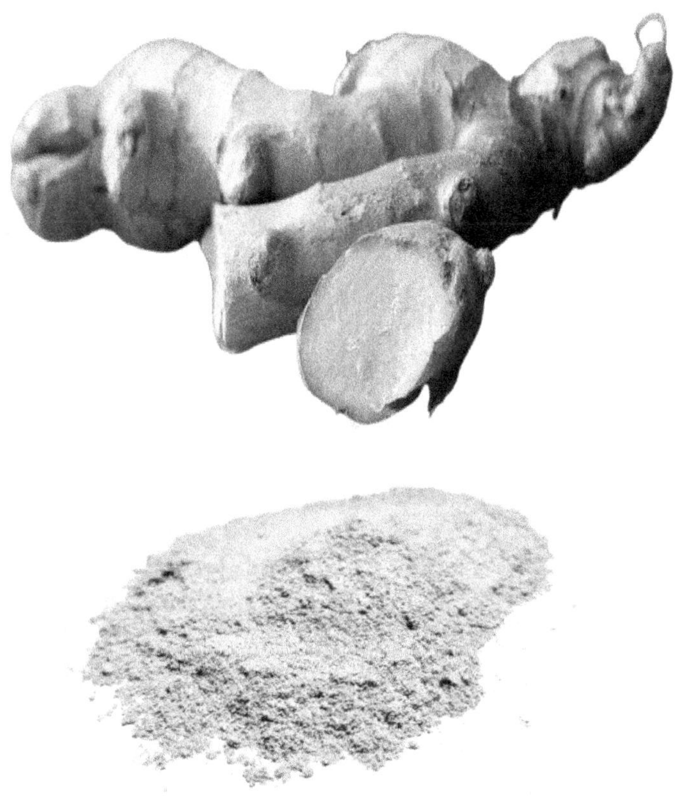

Vitamins & Minerals: Contains various bioactive compounds but limited vitamin content.

Benefits: Ginseng is often used for its energy enhancing properties; however, pregnant women should consult healthcare providers before use due to potential hormonal effects.

In summary

These herbs offer various nutritional benefits that can support expectant mothers throughout their pregnancy journey. However, it is essential to consult healthcare providers before using any herbal remedies to ensure safety and appropriateness for individual health needs. By understanding the nutritional profiles of these herbs, women can make informed choices that enhance their overall wellbeing during this transformative time.

How to Source Quality Herbs

To source quality herbs effectively, it is essential to consider several factors that ensure the herbs you purchase are safe, potent, and beneficial. Here's a guide on how to source quality herbs based on the search results.

1.Choose the Right Herb

 Research or consult with a qualified herbal practitioner to determine which herb is suitable for your needs. Different parts of the plant may have varying therapeutic effects, so knowing which part to use is crucial.

2.Check Growing Conditions

Ensure that the herbs are organically grown or sustainably wildcrafted from areas free of contaminants. Look for certifications such as USDA organic or other commitments to chemical free agriculture. This helps avoid exposure to pesticides, herbicides, and other harmful chemicals.

3.Assess Purity and Contamination

Be aware that some herbal products may contain contaminants such as heavy metals, pesticides, or undeclared substances. For purity and safety look for brand that conduct third party test.

4.Select Reputable Companies

Purchase herbs from well established companies with a good reputation. Research their sourcing practices and commitment to quality. High quality products often come from companies that prioritize ethical harvesting and sustainable practices.

5.Evaluate Preparation Methods

Different herbal preparations (teas, tinctures, capsules) can vary in potency and effectiveness. Ensure that the preparation method is appropriate for the herb you are using and that it preserves the active compounds.

6.Examine Freshness

Freshness is key to potency. Purchase dried herbs from suppliers with high turnover rates to ensure you're getting fresh products. Check expiration dates and avoid products that have been sitting on shelves for extended periods.

7.Trust Your Senses

When selecting dried herbs, use your senses to evaluate quality. High quality herbs should resemble their fresh counterparts in color, texture, fragrance, and taste.

8.Understand Shelf Life

Different herbal preparations have varying shelf lives. For example, tinctures can last longer due to their alcohol content, while dried leaves may only be viable for about a year. Be mindful of storage conditions to maintain potency.

9.Consult Local Herbalists

Engaging with local herbalists can provide valuable insights into sourcing quality herbs. Many herbal practitioners create small batches of remedies and can guide you on the best brands or sources for specific herbs.

10.Look for Certifications

 Seek out products that have been certified by reputable organizations in your various country (e.g., U.S. Pharmacopeia or NSF International) for quality assurance.

11.Beware of Adulteration

Some herbal products may be adulterated with cheaper substitutes or fillers that dilute their effectiveness. Always check ingredient lists carefully.

12. Consider Ethical Sourcing

Support brands that practice sustainable harvesting methods and ethical sourcing of their herbs.

13. Stay Informed About Regulations

Be aware that herbal supplements are not as strictly regulated as pharmaceuticals in many countries, including the U.S., which can affect product quality.

14. Educate Yourself on Herb Interactions

Understand potential interactions between herbs and medications you may be taking, as some herbs can affect drug efficacy or cause adverse effects.

15. Utilize Online Resources

Use reputable online resources and databases to research specific herbs, their uses, and any safety concerns associated with them.

By following these guidelines, you can enhance your ability to source high quality herbs that will support your health and wellness effectively while ensuring safety during use. Always consult healthcare professionals when incorporating new herbal remedies into your routine, especially during pregnancy or when managing specific health conditions.

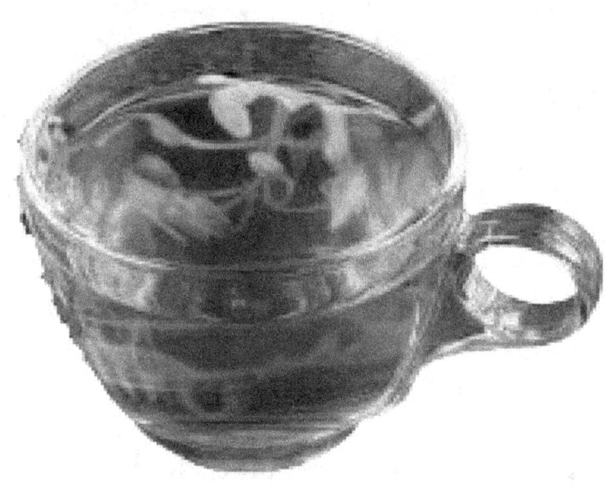

CHAPTER 3

HERBAL RECIPES FOR COMMON PREGNANCY DISCOMFORTS

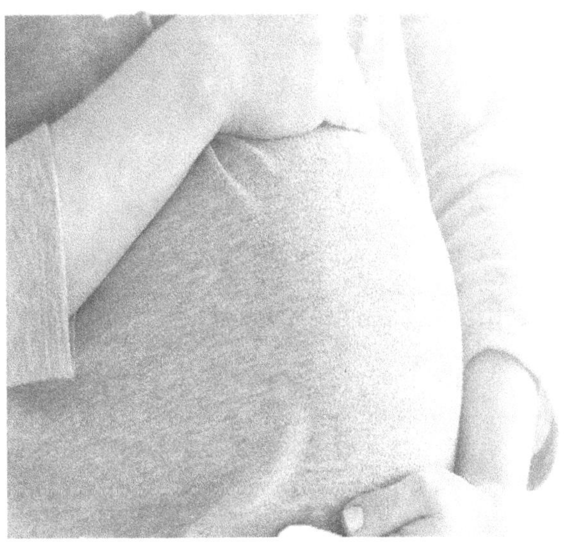

During pregnancy, many women experience a variety of discomforts due to the significant physical and hormonal changes occurring in their bodies. Understanding these common discomforts and their underlying reasons can help expectant mothers manage them more effectively. Here's an overview of some of the most prevalent pregnancy discomforts and the reasons behind them.

Common Pregnancy Discomforts and Their Reasons

1. Nausea and Vomiting (Morning Sickness)

Many pregnant women experience nausea and vomiting, particularly during the first trimester. This condition, often referred to as morning sickness, is thought to be caused by hormonal changes, particularly increased levels of human chorionic gonadotropin (HCG) and estrogen. Other contributing factors may include heightened sensitivity to smells and changes in digestion.

2. Constipation

Constipation is common during pregnancy due to increased levels of progesterone, which relaxes the muscles in the gastrointestinal tract, slowing down digestion. Additionally, the growing uterus exerts pressure on the intestines, further contributing to this discomfort. Iron supplements, often prescribed to prevent anemia, can exacerbate constipation.

3. Heartburn and Indigestion

As the uterus expands, it can push against the stomach, causing acid reflux and heartburn. Hormonal changes also slow down digestion, leading to increased acid production in the stomach. Foods that are spicy or high in fat can worsen these symptoms.

4. Backache

Back pain is common due to the additional weight gained during pregnancy and changes in posture as the body adapts to accommodate a growing fetus.

The loosening of ligaments due to hormonal changes can also contribute to back discomfort.

5. Fatigue

Fatigue is prevalent, especially during the first trimester and later stages of pregnancy. The body is working harder to support fetal growth, leading to increased energy expenditure. Hormonal fluctuations, particularly elevated progesterone levels, can also contribute to feelings of tiredness.

6. Dizziness

Dizziness or lightheadedness may occur due to low blood sugar levels or sudden changes in position (orthostatic hypotension). Increased blood volume during pregnancy can also lead to fluctuations in blood pressure.

7. Swelling (Edema)

Mild swelling of the hands and feet is common as pregnancy progresses. This is caused by increased blood volume and fluid retention due to hormonal changes. The growing uterus can also compress blood vessels in the pelvis, impeding circulation.

8. Leg Cramps

Leg cramps often occur at night and are thought to be related to changes in circulation and pressure from the growing uterus on nerves and blood vessels. Dehydration or low levels of certain minerals like calcium or magnesium may also contribute.

9. Breast Changes

Breast tenderness, swelling, and changes in size are common as hormonal levels rise in preparation for breastfeeding. The increase in fat tissue and milk glands can lead to discomfort as well.

10. Headaches

Headaches are common during pregnancy due to hormonal fluctuations, stress, fatigue, or dehydration. Changes in blood volume can also trigger headaches for some women.

11. Frequent Urination

Increased frequency of urination is common due to hormonal changes that increase blood flow to the kidneys as well as pressure from the growing uterus on the bladder.

12. Hemorrhoids

Hemorrhoids are swollen veins in the rectal area that can occur due to increased blood volume and pressure from the growing uterus on pelvic veins. Constipation can exacerbate this condition.

Understanding these common pregnancy discomforts helps expectant mothers recognize what they might experience throughout their journey. While many discomforts are a normal part of pregnancy, it's important for women to communicate with their healthcare providers about any severe or persistent symptoms that may require attention or intervention. By addressing these issues proactively, pregnant women can enhance their comfort and wellbeing during this transformative time.

Herbal Recipes for Common Pregnancy Discomforts

Here's an expanded list of herbal recipes for common pregnancy discomforts, each recipe targets specific issues that pregnant women may face.

Morning Sickness Remedies

1. Ginger Tea Recipe

Ginger is widely recognized for its ability to alleviate nausea and vomiting, making it an excellent remedy for morning sickness.

Ingredients:

4 cups filtered water

3.5 oz fresh ginger root, chopped (optionally peeled)

1 lemon, sliced

Honey (optional, to taste)

Instructions:

- Clean and chop the fresh ginger into 12inch pieces.

- In a small saucepan, bring the water to a boil over medium high heat.

- Add the chopped ginger and lemon slices to the boiling water.

- Reduce the heat to low and let it simmer for about 1015 minutes (longer for a stronger flavor).

Strain the tea into mugs and add honey if desired. Stir well and enjoy warm.

2. Peppermint Infusion Recipe

Peppermint can help soothe the stomach and reduce feelings of nausea.

Ingredients:

 1 tablespoon dried peppermint leaves (or a handful of fresh leaves)

 2 cups boiling water

Instructions:

- Place the peppermint leaves in a teapot or heatproof container.
- Pour boiling water over the leaves and steep for about 10 minutes.
- Strain the infusion into a cup and enjoy warm or cold.

- Drink this infusion after meals to help alleviate nausea and digestive discomfort.

Fatigue and Energy Boosters

3. Ginseng Tonic Recipe

Ginseng is known for its energy boosting properties, which can help combat fatigue during pregnancy.

Ingredients:

1 tablespoon ginseng root (dried or fresh)

4 cups water

Honey or lemon (optional)

Instructions:

- In a saucepan, bring the water to a boil.
- Add the ginseng root and reduce the heat to let it simmer for about 1520 minutes.
- Strain the tonic into a mug and add honey or lemon if desired.

- Enjoy this tonic once daily to help boost energy levels.

4. Herbal Smoothie Recipe

An herbal smoothie can provide a nutritious energy boost while incorporating various beneficial ingredients.

Ingredients:

1 banana

1 cup spinach

1 tablespoon moringa powder (or another nutrient rich powder)

1 cup almond milk or yogurt

Honey or maple syrup (optional)

Instructions:

- Combine all ingredients in a blender.
- Blend until smooth.

- Taste and adjust sweetness with honey or maple syrup if desired.
- Enjoy this smoothie as a nutritious breakfast or snack to help combat fatigue.

5. Lemon Balm Tea for Anxiety Relief

Lemon balm is known for its calming effects, which can help reduce anxiety during pregnancy.

Ingredients:

1 tablespoon dried lemon balm leaves

2 cups boiling water

Instructions:

- Steep lemon balm leaves in boiling water for about 10 minutes.
- Strain and enjoy warm or chilled.
- Drink this tea as needed to promote relaxation.

6. Oat Straw Infusion for Stress Relief

Oat straw is rich in nutrients and can help soothe nerves.

Ingredients:

2 tablespoons dried oat straw

4 cups boiling water

Instructions:

- Place oat straw in a heatproof container.
- Pour boiling water over it and steep for at least 30 minutes.
- Strain and drink throughout the day.

7. Fennel Seed Tea for Digestive Comfort

Fennel seeds can help relieve bloating and gas.

Ingredients:

1 teaspoon fennel seeds

1 cup boiling water

Instructions:

- Crush fennel seeds lightly to release their oils.
- Steep in boiling water for about 10 minutes.
- Strain and drink after meals.

8. Nettle Infusion for Nutritional Support

Nettle is rich in vitamins and minerals beneficial during pregnancy.

Ingredients:

1 tablespoon dried nettle leaves

2 cups boiling water

Instructions:

Steep nettle leaves in boiling water for about 10–15 minutes.

Strain and drink warm or cold once daily.

9. Red Raspberry Leaf Tea for Uterine Health

Red raspberry leaf is traditionally used to tone the uterus.

Ingredients:

 1 tablespoon dried red raspberry leaves

 1 cup boiling water

Instructions:

- Steep red raspberry leaves in boiling water for about 10 minutes.
- Strain and enjoy this tea once daily, particularly in the second trimester.

10. Clary Sage Tea for Hormonal Balance

Clary sage may help balance hormones during pregnancy.

Ingredients:

 1 teaspoon dried clary sage leaves

1 cup boiling water

Instructions:

- Steep clary sage leaves in boiling water for about 5–10 minutes.
- Strain and drink cautiously; consult your healthcare provider before use.

11. Valerian Root Tea for Sleep Support

Valerian root is known for its calming effects that promote sleep.

Ingredients:

1 teaspoon dried valerian root

1 cup boiling water

Instructions:

- Steep valerian root in boiling water for about 10 minutes.

- Strain and drink before bedtime to promote relaxation.

12. Hibiscus Tea for Hydration

Hibiscus tea is refreshing and helps maintain hydration.

Ingredients:

1 tablespoon dried hibiscus flowers

2 cups boiling water

Instructions:

- Steep hibiscus flowers in boiling water for about 10 minutes.
- Strain, cool, and serve over ice with a slice of lime if desired.

13. Catnip Tea for Relaxation

Catnip can help reduce stress and promote sleep.

Ingredients:

2 teaspoons dried catnip leaves

1 cup boiling water

Instructions:

- Steep catnip leaves in boiling water for about 5–10 minutes.
- Strain and enjoy before bedtime.

14. Cinnamon Infused Water for Blood Sugar Regulation

Cinnamon may help regulate blood sugar levels during pregnancy.

Ingredients:

1 cinnamon stick

4 cups of water

Instructions:

- Boil water with a cinnamon stick added.

- Let it steep until cooled; remove the stick before drinking.

Important Considerations

While these herbal remedies can provide relief from common pregnancy discomforts, it is crucial to consult with a healthcare provider before incorporating any new herbs or supplements into your routine, especially during pregnancy, as some herbs may have contraindications or may not be suitable during certain stages of pregnancy.

By utilizing these herbal recipes thoughtfully, expectant mothers can find natural ways to alleviate discomfort while supporting their overall health during this transformative time in their lives.

CHAPTER 4

NOURISHING HERBAL RECIPES

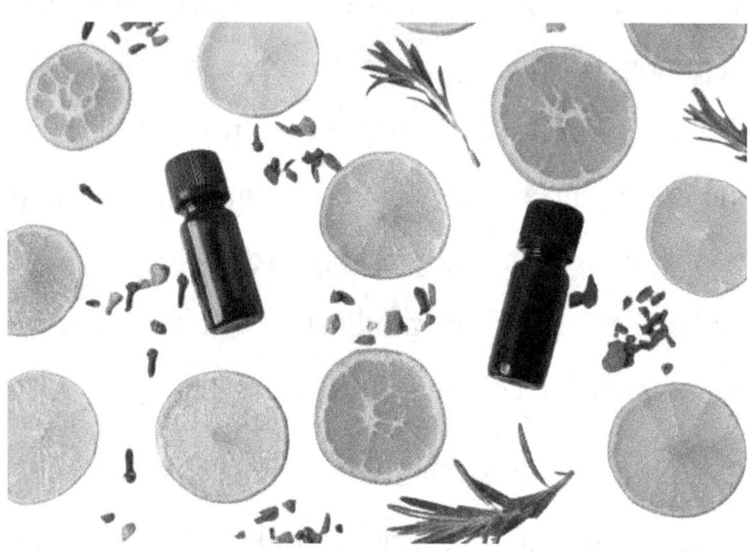

Nourishing herbal recipes are culinary creations that incorporate herbs known for their health benefits, providing both flavor and nutrition. These recipes not only enhance the taste of meals but also promote overall wellbeing by utilizing the medicinal properties of various herbs. The concept of nourishing herbal recipes emphasizes the importance of using whole, natural ingredients that support bodily functions, boost immunity, and contribute to a healthy lifestyle.

1. Understanding Nourishing Herbs

Nourishing herbs are plants that offer significant health benefits due to their rich nutritional profiles and therapeutic properties. They can be used in various forms, including fresh, dried, powdered, or as extracts. These herbs often contain vitamins, minerals, antioxidants, and other beneficial compounds that can help alleviate common ailments and enhance overall health.

For example:

Ginger is known for its antinausea properties and can aid digestion.

Peppermint is soothing for the digestive system and can relieve headaches.

Chamomile is recognized for its calming effects and can promote better sleep.

Incorporating these herbs into daily meals can create a holistic approach to nutrition, supporting both physical and mental health.

Nutrient Rich Herbal Broths

Nutrient rich herbal broths are flavorful liquids made by simmering various herbs, vegetables, and sometimes animal bones or mushrooms in water. These broths serve as a nourishing base for soups, stews, sauces, and grains, while also providing numerous health benefits. They are particularly valued for their ability to enhance digestion, support the immune system, and provide essential vitamins and minerals.

Benefits of Herbal Broths

1. Nutritional Powerhouse: Herbal broths are rich in vitamins, minerals, and antioxidants. When simmered, the nutrients from the herbs and vegetables leach into the broth, creating a nutrient dense liquid that can support overall health.

2. Digestive Support: The gelatin and amino acids released from bones (if used) help to soothe the digestive tract and may aid in healing gut related issues. Herbal ingredients like ginger and garlic can further enhance digestive health.

3. Immune Boosting: Many herbs used in broths have antimicrobial and antiinflammatory properties that can help strengthen the immune system. Ingredients like oregano, thyme, and rosemary have been shown to possess these beneficial qualities.

4. Hydration: Herbal broths provide a hydrating option that can be consumed alone or used as a base

for other dishes. Staying hydrated is crucial during pregnancy or when recovering from illness.

5. Flavor Enhancer: Beyond their health benefits, herbal broths add depth of flavor to various dishes. They can be used to cook grains like rice or quinoa, enhancing the taste while providing additional nutrients.

How to Make Nutrient Rich Herbal Broths

Creating your own herbal broth is simple and allows for flexibility based on personal taste preferences and available ingredients. Here's a basic guide along with some recipe ideas:

Basic Herbal Broth Recipe

Ingredients:

1 onion, quartered

23 carrots, chopped

23 celery stalks, chopped

4 cloves garlic, smashed

A handful of fresh herbs (e.g., parsley, thyme, rosemary)

Optional: 1 cup mushrooms (for umami flavor)

Salt and pepper to taste

Water (enough to cover ingredients)

Instructions:

- In a large pot, combine all the vegetables and herbs.
- Add enough water to cover the ingredients.

- Bring to a boil over medium high heat.

- Reduce heat and let it simmer for at least 30 minutes to 1 hour (the longer it simmers, the more flavorful it will be).

- Strain the broth through a fine mesh sieve or cheesecloth into another pot or container.

- Season with salt and pepper to taste.

- Store in airtight containers in the refrigerator for up to 4 days or freeze for longer storage.

Recipe Variations

Here are some variations of herbal broths that incorporate specific herbs known for their health benefits:

1. Immune Boosting Garden Herb Stock

Ingredients: Oregano, rosemary, sage, thyme, garlic, onion.

Benefits: These herbs are known for their antimicrobial properties and can help support immune function.

2. Nourishing Bone Broth

Ingredients: Animal bones (chicken or beef), apple cider vinegar (to extract minerals), carrots, celery, onion.

Benefits: Rich in collagen and amino acids that promote joint health and gut healing.

3. Vegan Herbal Broth

Ingredients: Seaweed (kombu or dulse), mushrooms (shiitake or reishi), ginger, garlic.

Benefits: Provides umami flavor while being nutrient dense and suitable for vegans.

4. Asian Inspired Herbal Broth

Ingredients: Ginger slices, garlic cloves, scallions, shiitake mushrooms, star anise.

Benefits: This broth can enhance digestion and provide warming properties.

Tips for Making Nutrient Rich Herbal Broths

1. Use Fresh Ingredients: Fresh herbs and vegetables will yield the best flavor and nutritional benefits.

2. Experiment with Herbs: Feel free to add different herbs based on your preferences or what you have available. Stinging nettles and oat straw are excellent additions for their vitamin rich qualities.

3. Save Kitchen Scraps: Use vegetable scraps like onion peels, carrot tops, or celery leaves to minimize waste while adding flavor to your broth.

4. Adjust Seasoning After Cooking: Taste your broth before serving; adjust seasoning as needed since flavors can intensify during cooking.

5. Store Properly: Always let your broth cool completely before storing it in airtight containers in the fridge or freezer.

Nutrient rich herbal broths are versatile culinary staples that offer numerous health benefits while enhancing the flavor of meals. By incorporating a variety of herbs and vegetables into your broths, you can create nourishing liquids that support overall wellbeing. Whether enjoyed on their own as a comforting drink or used as a base for soups and stews, herbal broths are a simple yet powerful addition to any diet.

Vegetable and Herb Broth Recipe

Vegetable and herb broth is a versatile culinary staple that can be used in various dishes or enjoyed on its own. This broth is packed with nutrients, flavor, and the health benefits of fresh herbs and vegetables. It's an excellent option for vegetarians and vegans, providing a rich, savory base without animal products.

Ingredients

Base Vegetables:

2 medium onions, quartered (skin on for added flavor)

3 carrots, chopped

3 celery stalks, chopped

4 cloves garlic, smashed

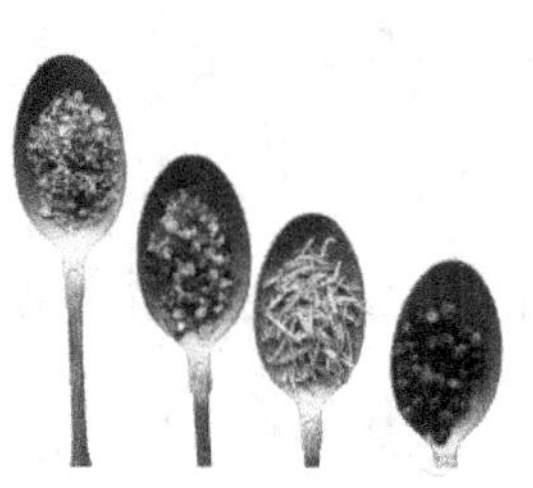

Herbs:

1 cup fresh parsley (stems included)

23 sprigs fresh thyme (or 1 tablespoon dried thyme)

2 sprigs fresh rosemary (or 1 tablespoon dried rosemary)

2 bay leaves

Additional Flavor Enhancers:

Optional: 1 cup mushrooms (shiitake or button) for umami flavor

Optional: A piece of kombu seaweed for added minerals

Seasoning:

Salt and pepper to taste

Water:

Approximately 12 cups of water (enough to cover the ingredients)

Instructions

1. Prepare the Ingredients:

Clean and chop the vegetables into large chunks. There's no need to peel the onions or garlic; the skins can add extra flavor and nutrients to the broth.

2. Combine Ingredients in a Pot:

In a large stockpot, combine the chopped onions, carrots, celery, garlic, parsley, thyme, rosemary, bay leaves, and any optional ingredients like mushrooms or kombu.

3. Add Water:

Pour in enough water to cover all the ingredients by about an inch (approximately 12 cups).

4. Bring to a Boil:

Place the pot over medium high heat and bring the mixture to a boil.

5. Simmer:

Once boiling, reduce the heat to low and let it simmer uncovered for about 45 minutes to an hour. This allows the flavors to meld together.

6. Strain the Broth:

After simmering, remove the pot from heat. Use a fine mesh strainer or cheesecloth to strain out the solids from the liquid broth. Discard the solids or compost them.

7. Season:

Taste the broth and season with salt and pepper as desired. You can also add a splash of apple cider vinegar for additional flavor and health benefits.

8. Cool and Store:

Allow the broth to cool before transferring it into airtight containers. Store in the refrigerator for up to one week or freeze for longer storage (up to six months). If freezing, leave some space at the top of containers to allow for expansion.

Serving Suggestions

As a Soup Base: Use this broth as a base for soups by adding cooked grains, beans, or additional vegetables.

Flavoring Grains: Cook rice, quinoa, or pasta in this broth instead of water for added flavor.

Sipping Broth: Enjoy a warm mug of broth on its own as a comforting drink.

Nutritional Benefits

This vegetable and herb broth is not only flavorful but also rich in nutrients from various vegetables and herbs. It provides vitamins A, C, K, and several B vitamins along with minerals such as potassium and magnesium. The herbs contribute antioxidants that can help support immune function and overall health.

Making your own vegetable and herb broth is an easy way to enhance your meals while ensuring you're consuming nutritious ingredients. This recipe is highly customizable; feel free to experiment with different herbs or vegetables based on your preferences or what you have on hand.

Enjoy this nourishing broth as part of your culinary repertoire.

Bone Broth with Herbs Recipe

Bone broth is a nutrient dense liquid made by simmering animal bones and connective tissues in water. It is rich in collagen, gelatin, amino acids, and minerals that support overall health. Adding herbs enhances the flavor and provides additional health benefits, making this broth not only delicious but also therapeutic.

Ingredients

Bones:

24 pounds of animal bones (chicken, beef, lamb, or pork)

Vegetables:

2 medium onions, quartered

3 carrots, chopped

3 celery stalks, chopped

4 cloves garlic, smashed

Herbs:

46 sprigs of fresh parsley (or 1 tablespoon dried)

23 sprigs fresh thyme (or 1 tablespoon dried)

2 sprigs fresh rosemary (or 1 tablespoon dried)

2 bay leaves

Flavor Enhancers:

¼ cup apple cider vinegar (to help extract minerals from the bones)

Water:

Approximately 12 cups of water (enough to cover the ingredients)

Instructions

1. Prepare the Bones:

If using raw bones, you can roast them in the oven at 400°F (200°C) for about 30 minutes until browned. This step adds depth of flavor to the broth.

2. Combine Ingredients in a Pot:

In a large stockpot or slow cooker, add the bones, chopped vegetables (onions, carrots, celery), smashed garlic cloves, and herbs (parsley, thyme, rosemary, bay leaves).

3. Add Vinegar and Water:

Pour in the apple cider vinegar and enough water to cover all the ingredients by about an inch (approximately 12 cups). The vinegar helps leach minerals from the bones.

4. Bring to a Boil:

Place the pot over medium high heat and bring the mixture to a boil.

5. Simmer:

Once boiling, reduce the heat to low and let it simmer uncovered for at least 12 hours (up to 24 hours for chicken bones; longer for beef bones). The longer it simmers, the more flavorful and nutrient rich it will become.

6. Strain the Broth:

After simmering, remove the pot from heat. Use a fine mesh strainer or cheesecloth to strain out the solids from the liquid broth. Discard the solids (bones and vegetables).

7. Cool and Store:

Allow the broth to cool slightly before transferring it into airtight containers. Store in the refrigerator for up to one week or freeze for longer storage (up to six months). If freezing, leave some space at the top of containers to allow for expansion.

8. Season Before Use:

When ready to use your bone broth, taste it and season with salt and pepper as desired.

Nutritional Benefits

Bone broth is known for its numerous health benefits:

Rich in Nutrients: Provides collagen and gelatin that support joint health and skin elasticity.

Gut Health: Contains amino acids like glycine and proline that promote gut healing.

Immune Support: Nutrient dense broth can help strengthen the immune system.

Hydration: A warm cup of bone broth is hydrating and comforting.

This bone broth with herbs recipe is not only simple to make but also provides a nourishing addition to your diet. Whether sipped on its own or used as a base for other dishes, this broth offers a wealth of flavor and health benefits. Experiment with different herbs or additional ingredients based on your preferences or seasonal availability to create your perfect bone broth.

Herbal Infused Oils and Salves

Herbal infused oils and salves are versatile preparations that combine the therapeutic properties of herbs with carrier oils, creating nourishing products for skin care, hair care, and culinary uses. These infused oils can be used in various applications, from topical treatments for skin conditions to flavorful additions in cooking. Below is a detailed exploration of herbal infused oils and salves, including how to make them and their benefits

Herbal Infused Oils and Salves

What Are Herbal Infused Oils?

Herbal infused oils are created by steeping herbs in a carrier oil, allowing the beneficial compounds of the herbs to be extracted into the oil. This process captures the healing properties of the herbs, making them available for use in various applications. Common carrier oils include olive oil, coconut oil, almond oil, and jojoba oil.

Benefits of Herbal Infused Oils

1. Skin Nourishment: Herbal infused oils can hydrate and soothe the skin, helping to reduce dryness, redness, and irritation. They can be particularly beneficial for conditions like eczema or psoriasis.

2. Anti-inflammatory Properties: Many herbs used in these infusions possess antiinflammatory properties that can help alleviate pain and swelling when applied topically.

3. Aromatherapy: The scents of infused oils can promote relaxation and reduce stress. Essential oils from herbs like lavender or chamomile offer calming effects.

4. Culinary Uses: Infused oils can enhance the flavor of dishes when used in cooking or as dressings. They provide a unique twist to salads, marinades, and sauces.

5. Versatility: Herbal infused oils can be used as a base for making salves, lotions, and other body care products.

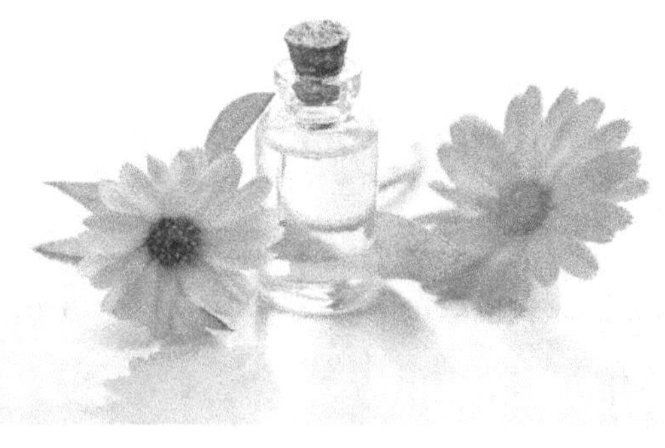

How to Make Herbal Infused Oils

There are two primary methods for making herbal infused oils: the cold infusion method and the heat infusion method.

Cold Infusion Method

This method allows for a gentle extraction of the herb's properties without heat.

Ingredients:

Dried herbs (e.g., calendula, lavender, rosemary)

Carrier oil (e.g., olive oil or almond oil)

Clean glass jar with a lid

Instructions:

Prepare Herbs: Use dried herbs to prevent moisture content from causing spoilage.

Fill Jar: Place the dried herbs in a clean glass jar, filling it about halfway.

Add Oil: Pour the carrier oil over the herbs until they are fully submerged.

Seal Jar: Close the jar tightly and place it in a cool, dark place.

Infusion Time: Let it sit for 46 weeks, shaking gently every few days to mix.

Strain Oil: After the infusion period, strain out the herbs using cheesecloth or a fine mesh strainer.

Store Oil: Transfer the infused oil into a clean bottle for storage.

Heat Infusion Method

This method speeds up the infusion process by using gentle heat.

Ingredients:

Dried herbs

Carrier oil

Double boiler or slow cooker.

Instructions:

- Prepare Herbs: Use dried herbs as before.

- Combine Ingredients: Place the dried herbs in a double boiler or slow cooker and cover them with carrier oil.

- Heat Gently: Heat on low for 24 hours (do not exceed 140°F/60°C) to avoid damaging the oil or herb properties.

- Strain Oil: After heating, strain out the herbs using cheesecloth or a fine mesh strainer.

- Store Oil: Transfer the infused oil into a clean bottle for storage.

Making Herbal Salves

Herbal salves are thicker preparations made by combining herbal infused oils with beeswax or another thickening agent.

Herbal Salve Recipe

Ingredients:

1 cup herbal infused oil (made using one of the methods above)

1/4 cup beeswax pellets (or more for a firmer salve)

Optional essential oils (e.g., tea tree or lavender) for added fragrance and benefits

Instructions:

- Melt Beeswax: In a double boiler, melt the beeswax over low heat until fully liquefied.
- Combine Oils: Add the herbal infused oil to the melted beeswax and stir well to combine.
- Add Essential Oils (Optional): If desired, add a few drops of essential oils at this stage for additional benefits.

- Pour into Containers: Quickly pour the mixture into small jars or tins before it begins to harden.

- Cool Completely: Allow salves to cool completely before sealing with lids.

- Store Properly: Store in a cool, dark place; salves typically last up to one year.

Herbal infused oils and salves provide an excellent way to harness the healing properties of plants while creating nourishing products for skin care and culinary use. By following simple methods to infuse herbs into carrier oils and then creating salves from those infusions, you can enjoy natural remedies that enhance your selfcare routines and culinary experiences.

CHAPTER 5

HERBAL TEAS FOR RELAXATION AND WELLNESS

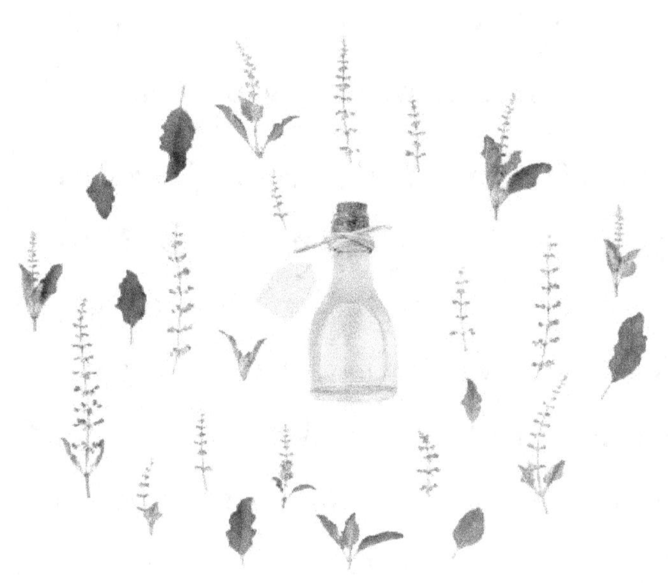

Herbal teas have long been celebrated for their calming effects and health benefits. These infusions of herbs, flowers, and other botanicals provide a natural way to promote relaxation and overall wellness. Below is a detailed overview of herbal teas specifically designed for relaxation and wellness, including some popular ingredients, their benefits, and how to prepare them.

Based on the provided search results, here's a categorization of herbal teas specifically focusing on Calming Herbal Teas and Teas for Digestive Health.

Calming Herbal Teas

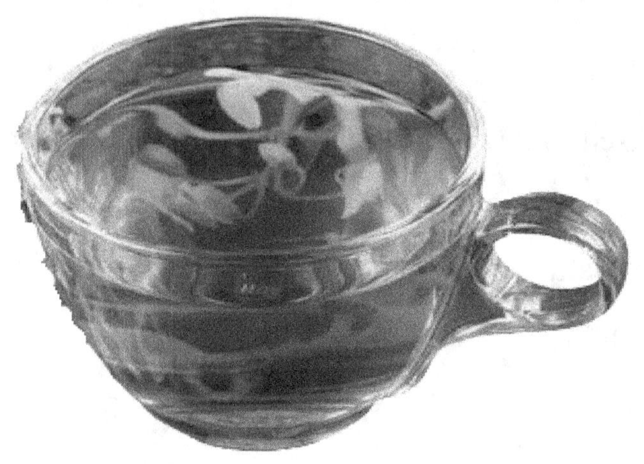

1. Chamomile Tea

Benefits:

Known for its mild sedative properties, chamomile helps reduce anxiety and promote sleep. It is often recommended for evening consumption to improve sleep quality.

Preparation:

Steep 12 teaspoons of dried chamomile flowers in hot water for about 510 minutes.

2. Lavender Tea

Benefits:

Lavender tea is famous for its calming aroma, which can help alleviate stress and anxiety. It is also effective in improving sleep quality.

Preparation:

Steep 12 teaspoons of dried lavender buds in hot water for 510 minutes.

3. Peppermint Tea

Benefits:

While primarily known for aiding digestion, peppermint tea also has calming effects that can relieve stress and tension.

Preparation:

Steep fresh or dried peppermint leaves in boiling water for 57 minutes.

4. Passionflower Tea

Benefits:

Passionflower is recognized for its ability to reduce anxiety and improve sleep quality by increasing levels of GABA in the brain.

Preparation:

Steep 1 teaspoon of dried passionflower in hot water for about 10 minutes.

5. Lemon Balm Tea

Benefits:

Lemon balm is known to reduce stress and anxiety, improve mood, and promote relaxation.

Preparation:

Steep 12 teaspoons of dried lemon balm leaves in hot water for 510 minutes.

6. Valerian Root Tea

Benefits:

Valerian root is often used as a natural sedative to help with insomnia and anxiety.

Preparation:

Steep 1 teaspoon of dried valerian root in hot water for about 10 minutes.

7. Holy Basil (Tulsi) Tea

Benefits:

Holy basil is an adaptogen that helps the body cope with stress and promotes mental clarity.

Preparation:

Steep fresh or dried holy basil leaves in hot water for about 510 minutes.

8. Rose Tea

Benefits:

Rose tea has calming properties that can help alleviate anxiety and promote relaxation while providing a pleasant floral flavor.

Preparation:

Steep dried rose petals in hot water for about 510 minutes.

Teas for Digestive Health

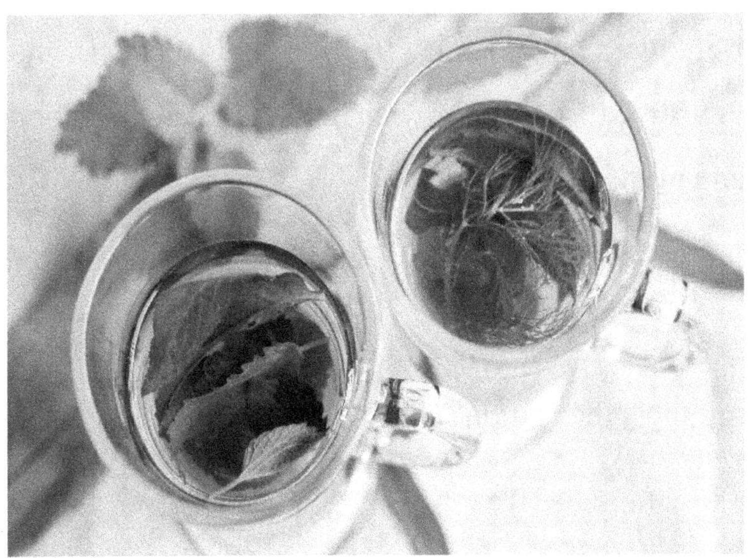

1. Peppermint Tea

Benefits: Known for its digestive benefits, peppermint tea can soothe upset stomachs, relieve gas, and reduce bloating.

Preparation:

Steep fresh or dried peppermint leaves in boiling water for 57 minutes.

2. Ginger Tea

Benefits: Ginger tea is effective against nausea and digestive discomfort. It can help stimulate digestion and alleviate bloating.

Preparation:

Boil sliced fresh ginger root in water for about 1015 minutes, then strain.

3. Fennel Seed Tea

Benefits:

Fennel seeds are known to aid digestion, reduce bloating, and relieve gas.

Preparation:

Crush fennel seeds lightly and steep them in boiling water for about 10 minutes.

4. Hawthorn Tea

Benefits:

While primarily known for heart health, hawthorn can also support digestive function by promoting healthy blood flow to the digestive organs.

Preparation:

Steep dried hawthorn berries in boiling water for about 10 minutes.

5. Rooibos Tea

Benefits: Naturally caffeine free, rooibos tea may help soothe digestive issues while providing antioxidants.

Preparation:

Brew rooibos tea bags or loose leaves in boiling water for about 5 minutes.

6. Lemon Balm Tea

Benefits: In addition to its calming effects, lemon balm can help alleviate digestive discomfort and improve overall gut health.

Preparation:

- Steep dried lemon balm leaves in hot water for 510 minutes.

Herbal teas serve as a natural remedy to promote relaxation and support digestive health. The calming herbal teas listed above are ideal for reducing stress and enhancing sleep quality, while the digestive health teas can alleviate gastrointestinal discomforts. Incorporating these herbal infusions into your daily routine can contribute significantly to overall wellness. Always consult with a healthcare provider before starting any new herbal regimen, especially if you have existing health conditions or are pregnant.

CHAPTER 6

SPECIAL CONSIDERATIONS BY TRIMESTER

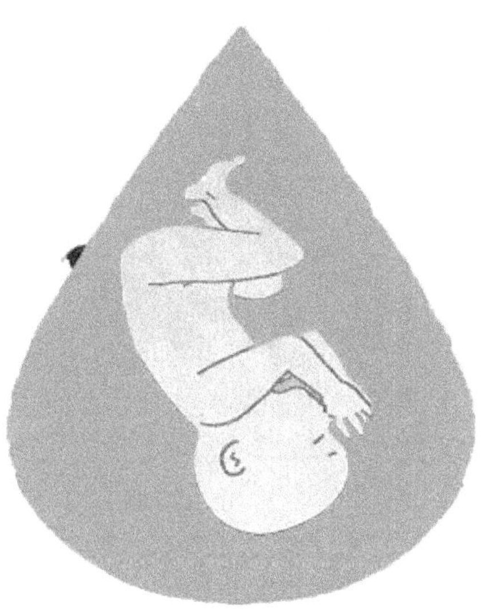

Pregnancy is divided into three trimesters, each with unique physiological changes and challenges. Understanding these changes can help expectant mothers make informed decisions about their health, including the use of herbal remedies. Below is an overview of special considerations for each trimester, focusing on safe herbs and practices.

First Trimester: Safe Herbs and Recipes

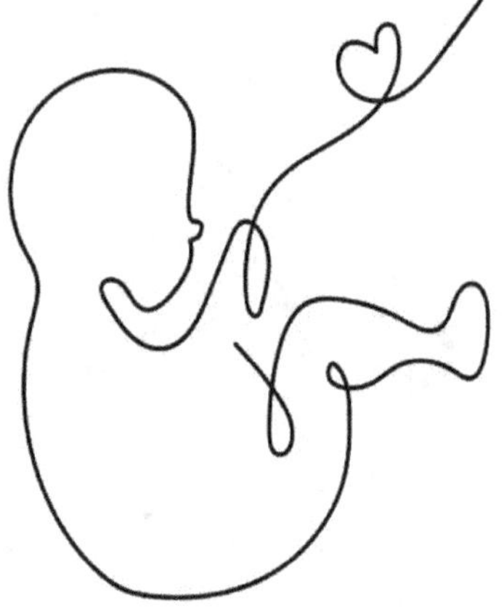

The first trimester (weeks 112) is a critical period for fetal development and often involves significant hormonal changes. Many women experience common discomforts such as nausea, fatigue, and mood swings. While some may seek relief through herbal remedies, it is essential to approach this with caution, as not all herbs are safe during pregnancy.

Below is an overview of safe herbs, their benefits, and recipes suitable for the first trimester.

Safe Herbs for the First Trimester

Ginger

Benefits: Ginger is widely recognized for its effectiveness in reducing nausea and vomiting, particularly morning sickness. It can also aid digestion and alleviate gastrointestinal discomfort.

Usage: Ginger tea or ginger ale can be consumed to alleviate nausea. A typical recipe includes steeping 12 teaspoons of fresh grated ginger in hot water for 10 minutes.

Peppermint

Benefits: Peppermint can help soothe digestive issues and relieve nausea. It may also reduce headaches and improve mood.

Usage: Peppermint tea can be made by steeping fresh or dried peppermint leaves in boiling water for 57 minutes. It can also be added to lemonade or used in cooking.

1. Chamomile

Benefits: Chamomile is known for its calming effects and can help with sleep disturbances and anxiety. It has mild antiinflammatory properties that may soothe the digestive system.

Usage: Chamomile tea can be enjoyed once or twice a day by steeping 12 teaspoons of dried chamomile flowers in hot water for 510 minutes.

2. Cranberry

Benefits: Cranberry juice is beneficial for preventing urinary tract infections (UTIs), which are common during pregnancy. It is rich in vitamin C and antioxidants.

Usage: Drinking unsweetened cranberry juice or making a homemade cranberry infusion can help maintain urinary health.

3. Red Raspberry Leaf

Benefits: Often recommended for later stages of pregnancy, red raspberry leaf is believed to tone the uterus and may help with nausea.

Usage: Consult a healthcare provider before using red raspberry leaf in the first trimester, as opinions vary on its safety during this period.

4. Lemon Balm

Benefits: Lemon balm has calming properties that can help reduce anxiety and improve sleep quality. It may also aid digestion.

Usage: Steep 12 teaspoons of dried lemon balm leaves in hot water for 510 minutes to make a soothing tea.

Recipes for the First Trimester

Here are some simple herbal recipes that incorporate the safe herbs listed above:

1. Ginger Tea Recipe

Ingredients:

12 inches fresh ginger root, sliced

2 cups water

Honey (optional)

Instructions:

- Boil the water in a saucepan.
- Add the sliced ginger and let it simmer for about 10 minutes.
- Strain into a cup and add honey if desired.
- Enjoy this tea to alleviate nausea.

2. Peppermint Tea Recipe

Ingredients:

1 tablespoon dried peppermint leaves (or a handful of fresh leaves)

2 cups boiling water

Instructions:

- Place peppermint leaves in a teapot.
- Pour boiling water over the leaves and steep for about 10 minutes.
- Strain and enjoy warm or cold after meals to reduce nausea.

3. Chamomile Tea Recipe

Ingredients:

1 tablespoon dried chamomile flowers

1 cup boiling water.

Instructions:

- Steep chamomile flowers in boiling water for about 510 minutes.
- Strain into a cup and enjoy before bedtime for relaxation.

4. Cranberry Infusion Recipe

Ingredients:

1 cup fresh cranberries (or unsweetened cranberry juice)

4 cups water

Instructions:

- If using fresh cranberries, boil them in water until they burst (about 10 minutes).
- Strain the mixture to extract the juice, adding honey for sweetness if desired.
- Consume daily to help prevent UTIs.

5. Lemon Balm Tea Recipe

Ingredients:

1 tablespoon dried lemon balm leaves

2 cups boiling water

Instructions:

- Steep lemon balm leaves in boiling water for about 10 minutes.
- Strain and enjoy warm or chilled to promote relaxation.

During the first trimester, it is crucial to prioritize safety when considering herbal remedies. The herbs listed above are generally regarded as safe when consumed in moderation, but it is always best to consult with a healthcare provider before incorporating any new herbs into your routine during pregnancy.

These herbal teas not only provide relief from common discomforts but also contribute to overall wellness during this important stage of pregnancy. By embracing these natural remedies, expectant mothers can support their health while nurturing their growing baby.

Second Trimester: Supporting Growth and Development

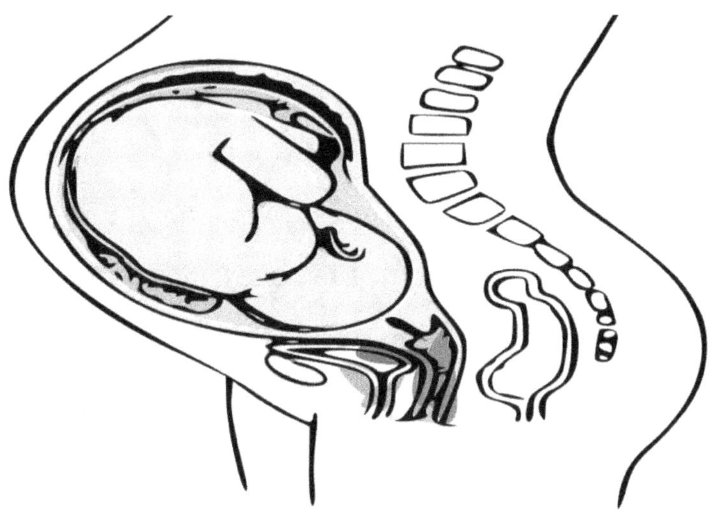

The second trimester of pregnancy, which spans from weeks 13 to 27, is often referred to as the "honeymoon phase" due to the reduction in nausea and fatigue that many women experiences. This period is characterized by significant fetal growth and development, as well as various physical and emotional changes for the mother. Here are some key considerations for supporting growth and development during this important stage of pregnancy.

Key Changes and Developments

1. Fetal Growth:

By the end of the second trimester, the fetus typically measures about 14 inches in length and weighs around two pounds. Major organs and systems continue to mature, and the baby begins to develop its own sleep wake cycles.

Movements become more noticeable, often referred to as "quickening," which usually occurs around 20 weeks.

2. Maternal Changes:

Many women experience increased energy levels and a decrease in morning sickness symptoms.

Physical changes include a growing belly, which may lead to stretch marks and skin changes. Some women may also experience swelling in the ankles or hands.

3. Hormonal Adjustments:

Hormonal levels continue to fluctuate, which can affect mood, appetite, and physical sensations. Increased blood volume may lead to dizziness or lightheadedness.

Supporting Growth and Development

To support both maternal health and fetal development during the second trimester, consider the following recommendations:

1. Nutrition:

Balanced Diet: Focus on a diet rich in fruits, vegetables, whole grains, lean proteins, and healthy fats. This provides essential nutrients for both mother and baby.

Increased Caloric Intake: Aim for an additional 300 calories per day to support fetal growth without overeating.

Hydration: Drink plenty of water to stay hydrated, which is crucial for maintaining amniotic fluid levels.

2. Prenatal Vitamins:

Continue taking prenatal vitamins that include folic acid, iron, calcium, and DHA to support fetal development and maternal health.

3. Regular Exercise:

Engage in light to moderate exercise such as walking, swimming, or prenatal yoga. Exercise can help alleviate discomfort, improve mood, and prepare the body for labor.

4. Routine Prenatal Care:

Attend regular prenatal visits every 24 weeks to monitor maternal health and fetal development. Your healthcare provider will check weight gain, blood pressure, and perform necessary screenings.

5. Education and Preparation:

Consider taking prenatal classes that cover childbirth preparation, breastfeeding, infant CPR, and parenting skills.

Begin planning for your baby's arrival by creating a nursery space and discussing parenting roles with your partner.

Safe Herbs for the Second Trimester

While many herbs are safe during pregnancy, it's essential to consult with a healthcare provider before using any herbal remedies. Here are some herbs that are generally considered safe during the second trimester:

1. Ginger: Helps alleviate nausea and supports digestion.

2. Peppermint: Soothes digestive discomfort and may relieve headaches.

3. Red Raspberry Leaf: Often recommended during this trimester to prepare the uterus for labor; consult a healthcare provider before use.

4. Chamomile: Provides calming effects; can help with sleep disturbances.

5. Lemon Balm: Known for its calming properties; helps reduce anxiety.

Recipes for the Second Trimester

Here are some nutritious recipes that incorporate safe ingredients beneficial during the second trimester:

1. Ginger Tea

Ingredients:

12 inches fresh ginger root, sliced

2 cups water

Honey (optional)

Instructions:

Boil water in a saucepan.

Add sliced ginger and simmer for about 10 minutes.

Strain into a cup; add honey if desired.

2. Peppermint Tea

Ingredients:

1 tablespoon dried peppermint leaves (or fresh)

2 cups boiling water

Instructions:

Place peppermint leaves in a teapot.

Pour boiling water over leaves; steep for about 10 minutes.

Strain and enjoy warm or cold.

3. Red Raspberry Leaf Tea

Ingredients:

1 tablespoon dried red raspberry leaves

1 cup boiling water

Instructions:

- Steep red raspberry leaves in boiling water for about 10 minutes.
- Strain and drink once daily.

Chamomile Tea

Ingredients:

1 tablespoon dried chamomile flowers

1 cup boiling water

Instructions:

- Steep chamomile flowers in boiling water for about 510 minutes.
- Strain into a cup; enjoy before bedtime.

5. Lemon Balm Tea

Ingredients:

1 tablespoon dried lemon balm leaves

2 cups boiling water

Instructions:

- Steep lemon balm leaves in boiling water for about 10 minutes.
- Strain and enjoy warm or chilled.

The second trimester is a vital period for both maternal wellbeing and fetal development. By focusing on proper nutrition, regular exercise, routine prenatal care, and safe herbal remedies, expectant mothers can support their health while nurturing their growing baby. It's important to remain informed about changes during this trimester and make proactive choices that contribute positively to pregnancy outcomes. Always consult with healthcare providers regarding any concerns or questions about herbal use or overall health during pregnancy.

Third Trimester: Preparing for Labor

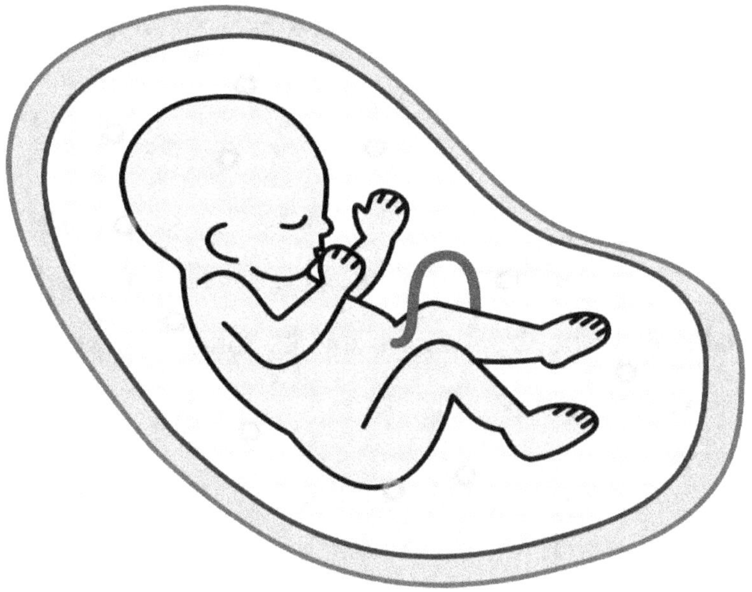

The third trimester of pregnancy, spanning from weeks 28 to 40, is a pivotal time as expectant mothers prepare for the arrival of their baby. This period is marked by significant physical and emotional changes, as well as the culmination of fetal development. Below are key considerations, symptoms, and preparations for labor during this important stage of pregnancy, along with nutritious recipes to support maternal health.

Key Changes and Developments

1. Fetal Growth:

By the end of the third trimester, the fetus typically measures about 19 to 21 inches long and weighs between 6 to 9 pounds.

The organs continue to mature, and the fetus gains more than half of its body weight during this period. It also begins to position itself head down in preparation for birth.

2. Maternal Changes:

Many women experience increased discomfort as the uterus expands and puts pressure on surrounding organs. Common symptoms include shortness of breath, frequent urination, backaches, and Braxton Hicks contractions (false labor).

Emotional fluctuations may occur as excitement about meeting the baby mixes with anxiety about labor and parenthood.

3. Healthcare Visits:

Prenatal visits become more frequent, typically every two weeks until week 36, then weekly until delivery. These visits include monitoring fetal growth, checking blood pressure, and performing necessary tests such as Group B strep screening.

Preparing for Labor

As the due date approaches, there are several important steps expectant mothers can take to prepare for labor:

1. Childbirth Education:

Consider enrolling in childbirth classes to learn about labor stages, pain management options, and what to expect during delivery.

2. Create a Birth Plan:

Draft a birth plan outlining preference for labor and delivery, including pain relief options, positions for labor, and who will be present during the birth.

3. Pack a Hospital Bag:

Prepare a hospital bag with essentials for both mother and baby. Include items such as comfortable clothing, toiletries, snacks, a camera or phone for photos, and items for the baby (e.g., outfits, blankets).

4. Monitor Fetal Movements:

Keep track of your baby's movements through kick counts. Familiarize yourself with your baby's patterns so you can notice any changes that may require medical attention.

5. Prepare the Nursery:

Set up a nursery or designated space for your newborn with essential items like a crib, diapers, clothes, and feeding supplies.

6. Discuss Postpartum Plans:

Consider discussing postpartum care with your healthcare provider. This includes plans for breastfeeding support, physical recovery after birth, and any mental health resources you may need.

7. Stay Active:

Engage in light exercise such as walking or prenatal yoga to help maintain strength and flexibility as you prepare for labor.

Safe Herbs for the Third Trimester

Several herbs are considered safe during the third trimester that can help prepare the body for labor:

Red Raspberry Leaf: Known for toning the uterus, it may help facilitate labor and reduce complications during delivery.

Ginger: Helpful for digestion; it can alleviate nausea if it persists.

Peppermint: Can relieve digestive discomforts such as gas or heartburn.

Chamomile: Offers calming effects that can help with sleep disturbances.

Lemon Balm: Known for its soothing properties that can reduce anxiety.

Recipes for the Third Trimester

Here are some nutritious recipes incorporating safe herbs beneficial during the third trimester:

1. Red Raspberry Leaf Tea

Ingredients:

1 tablespoon dried red raspberry leaves

1 cup boiling water

Instructions:

Steep red raspberry leaves in boiling water for about 10 minutes.

Strain into a cup; enjoy once daily to support uterine health.

2. Ginger Tea

Ingredients:

12 inches fresh ginger root, sliced

2 cups water

Honey (optional)

- Instructions:
- Boil water in a saucepan.
- Add sliced ginger and simmer for about 10 minutes.

- Strain into a cup; add honey if desired.

3. Peppermint Tea

Ingredients:

1 tablespoon dried peppermint leaves (or fresh)

2 cups boiling water

Instructions:

- Place peppermint leaves in a teapot.
- Pour boiling water over leaves; steep for about 10 minutes.
- Strain and enjoy warm or cold after meals.

4. Chamomile Tea

Ingredients:

1 tablespoon dried chamomile flowers

1 cup boiling water

Instructions:

- Steep chamomile flowers in boiling water for about 510 minutes.

- Strain into a cup; enjoy before bedtime for relaxation.

5. Lemon Balm Tea

Ingredients:

1 tablespoon dried lemon balm leaves

2 cups boiling water

Instructions:

- Steep lemon balm leaves in boiling water for about 10 minutes.

- Strain and enjoy warm or chilled to promote calmness.

The third trimester is a critical period of preparation for both labor and motherhood. By focusing on proper nutrition, hydration, regular exercise, safe herbal remedies, and education about childbirth, expectant mothers can support their health while preparing for their baby's arrival. Always consult with healthcare providers regarding any concerns or questions about herbal use or overall health during pregnancy to ensure a safe and healthy experience leading up to delivery.

The recommendations for safe herbs during pregnancy tend to remain consistent across trimesters due to their established safety profiles, traditional uses, and the emphasis on moderation. While some herbs may have specific applications in later stages of pregnancy, their overall benefits contribute to their inclusion in herbal remedies throughout all trimesters. Pregnant women should always consult with healthcare providers before using any herbal products to ensure safety tailored to their individual circumstances.

CHAPTER 7

CREATING YOUR OWN HERBAL REMEDIES

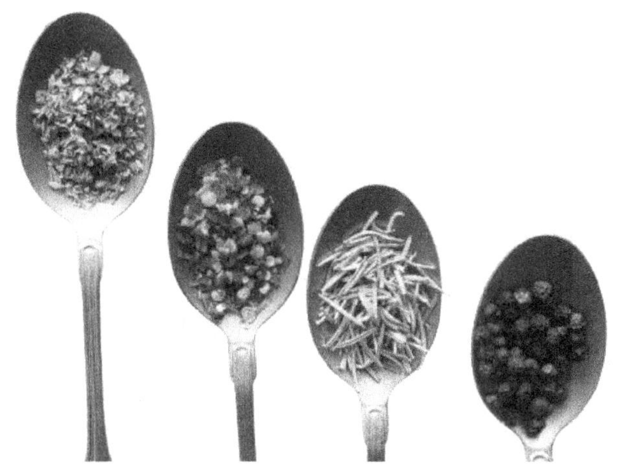

Creating your own herbal remedies is an empowering and rewarding practice that allows you to harness the healing properties of plants for personal use. Whether you're looking to make soothing teas, effective salves, or potent tinctures, understanding the basic techniques and tips for personalizing your recipes can enhance your experience and results.

Basic Techniques for Making Herbal Remedies

1. Understanding Herbal Preparations:

Teas: Herbal teas are one of the simplest forms of herbal remedies. They are made by steeping dried herbs in hot water, allowing the beneficial compounds to infuse into the liquid.

Tinctures: Tinctures are concentrated herbal extracts made by soaking herbs in alcohol or vinegar. This method extracts active components that may not dissolve in water.

Salves and Ointments: These topical preparations combine infused oils with a thickening agent like beeswax to create a soothing balm for skin issues.

2. Gathering Ingredients:

Use fresh or dried herbs based on availability. Dried herbs are often more potent and have a longer shelf life. Ensure you source high quality herbs from reputable suppliers or grow your own.

Commonly used herbs include chamomile (for relaxation), calendula (for skin healing), and ginger (for digestion).

3. Infusing Oils:

To make herbal infused oils, place dried herbs in a jar and cover them with a carrier oil (such as olive or almond oil). Allow the mixture to steep in a warm place for several days to extract the herb's properties.

For quicker results, use a double boiler method to gently heat the mixture for several hours.

4. Making Salves:

After creating an infused oil, melt beeswax in a double boiler, then mix in the infused oil until fully combined. Pour into containers and allow to cool.

The consistency can be adjusted by varying the amount of beeswax used.

5. Creating Tinctures:

Chop fresh herbs or coarsely grind dried herbs, then place them in a jar. Cover with alcohol (typically 80100 proof) or vinegar, seal tightly, and let steep for 46 weeks. Shake occasionally.

Strain the mixture through cheesecloth or a fine mesh strainer into dark glass bottles for storage.

Tips for Personalizing Your Recipes

1. Know Your Herbs:

Familiarize yourself with the properties of different herbs and how they interact with each other. Some herbs may have synergistic effects when combined, enhancing their overall benefits.

Consider your specific needs—whether it's stress relief, digestive support, or skin healing—and choose herbs accordingly.

2. Experiment with Ratios:

When creating blends (especially for teas), use parts to measure ingredients rather than fixed measurements. For example, you might use 2 parts chamomiles to 1part peppermint.

Start with small batches to test combinations and adjust ratios based on taste and effectiveness.

3. Incorporate Flavor Enhancers:

To improve the taste of your herbal remedies, consider adding flavor enhancing ingredients such as dried fruits (like apple or orange peel), spices (like cinnamon or ginger), or sweeteners (like honey).

This not only makes your remedies more enjoyable but can also add additional health benefits.

4. Document Your Creations:

Keep a journal of your recipes, noting down ingredients, ratios, preparation methods, and effects observed after use. This will help you refine your recipes over time.

Recording your process also allows you to replicate successful blends in the future.

5. Be Mindful of Safety:

Research any potential side effects or interactions between herbs and medications you may be taking.

Always perform a patch test when using new topical remedies to check for allergic reactions.

6. Engage Your Senses:

Use your senses when creating herbal remedies; observe colors, scents, and textures of the herbs you work with. This sensory engagement can enhance creativity and enjoyment in the process.

Creating your own herbal remedies is not only a practical skill but also a deeply rewarding experience that connects you with nature's healing potential. By mastering basic techniques and personalizing your recipes according to your needs and preferences, you can develop effective remedies that enhance your wellbeing. Whether you're crafting soothing teas for relaxation or nourishing salves for skin care, embracing this practice can lead to greater self-sufficiency and empowerment in managing health naturally.

CHAPTER 8

BONUSES

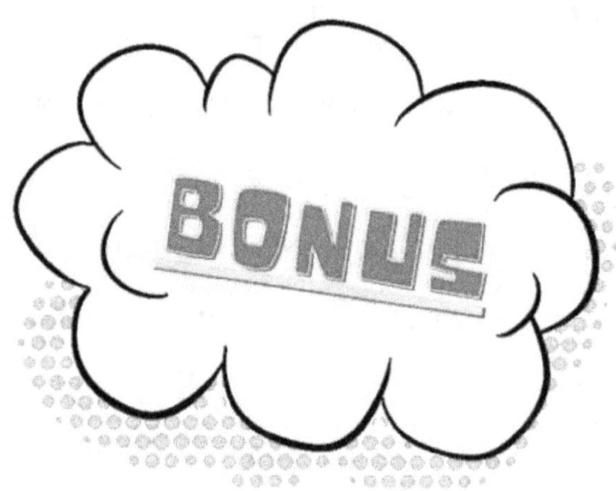

Positive affirmation cards

What Are Positive Affirmation Cards?

Positive affirmation cards are small, portable cards that feature uplifting statements designed to inspire and encourage positive thinking. Each card typically contains a concise affirmation written in the present tense, reflecting a desired state of being or a quality one wishes to embody. These cards serve as reminders of inner strength and resilience, helping individuals cultivate a positive mindset, especially during challenging times such as pregnancy.

Importance of Positive Affirmation Cards

1. Empowerment: During pregnancy, women often experience a range of emotions, including anxiety and self-doubt. Positive affirmations can empower expectant mothers by reinforcing their confidence in their bodies and their ability to navigate labor and delivery successfully.

2. Mental Well-being: Regularly using affirmation cards helps shift focus away from negative thoughts and fears. This practice can enhance mental well-being by promoting self-love, reducing stress, and fostering a sense of calmness.

3. Mindfulness: Incorporating affirmation cards into daily routines encourages mindfulness. By taking a moment to reflect on the affirmations, pregnant women can center themselves, connect with their bodies, and prepare mentally for childbirth.

4. Supportive Tool: Affirmation cards can be used alongside herbal remedies discussed in "Herbal Recipes for Pregnant women." While herbs may address physical discomforts, affirmations can help manage emotional challenges, creating a holistic approach to pregnancy wellness.

5. Daily Ritual: Establishing a daily ritual with affirmation cards can provide structure and consistency. Pregnant women can start or end their day by selecting an affirmation card, allowing them to set positive intentions for the day ahead or reflect on their journey.

Usage of Positive Affirmation Cards in Relation to the Book

1. Daily Practice: Readers can incorporate these affirmation cards into their daily routine by selecting one card each morning or evening. This practice encourages them to internalize the positive message and carry it throughout their day.

2. Visual Reminders: Affirmation cards can be placed in visible locations such as on mirrors, bedside tables, or inside birthing bags. This visibility serves as a constant reminder of their strength and capabilities as they approach labor.

3. Journaling Prompts: The affirmations can also serve as prompts for journaling. Readers can reflect on how each affirmation resonates with them or write about their feelings related to pregnancy and childbirth.

4. Sharing with Support Networks: Expectant mothers can share these cards with friends, family members, or support groups to foster a sense of community and encouragement during pregnancy.

5. Combining with Herbal Remedies: As readers explore herbal recipes for alleviating common pregnancy discomforts, they can pair these remedies with corresponding affirmations that promote relaxation and confidence in their body's ability to handle labor.

In "Herbal Recipes for Pregnant women," the inclusion of positive affirmation cards serves as a powerful tool for enhancing the overall experience of expectant mothers. By promoting empowerment, mental well-being, mindfulness, and daily structure, these affirmation cards complement the book's focus on herbal remedies, creating a holistic approach to pregnancy wellness that nurtures both body and mind.

Printable Positive affirmation templates

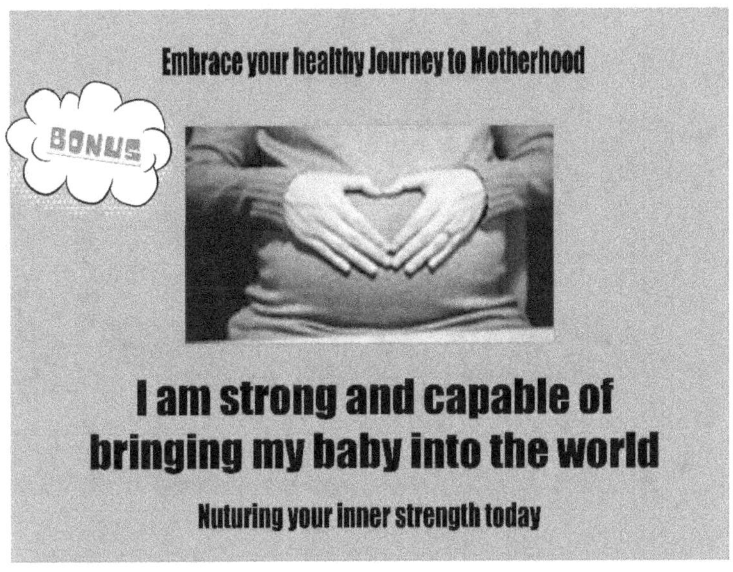

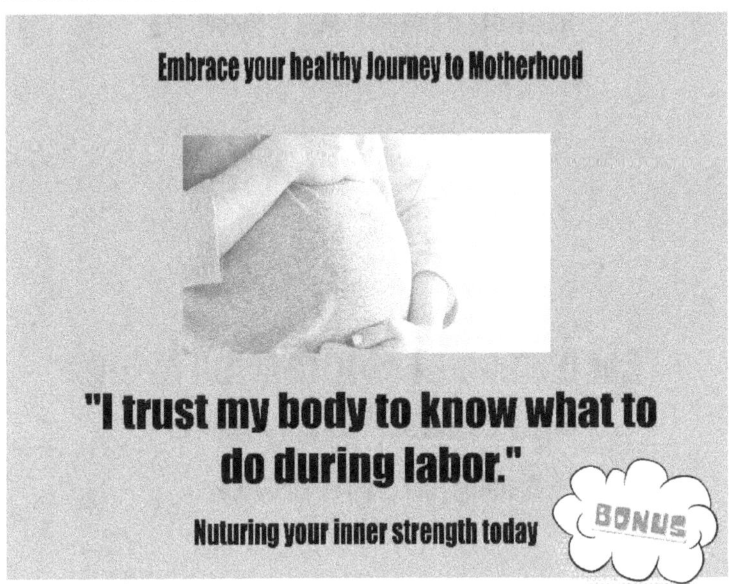

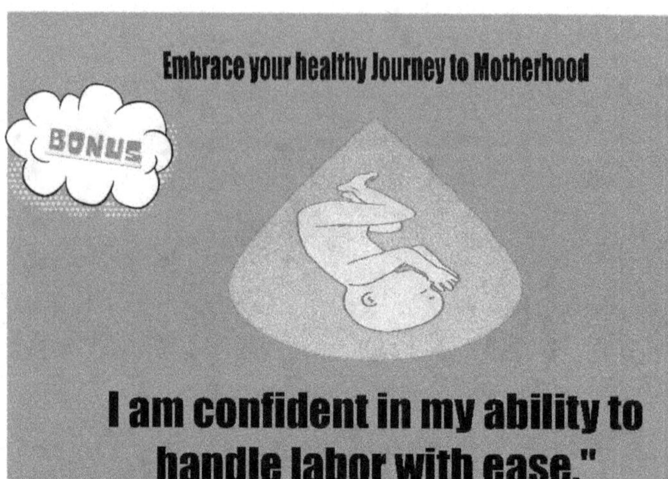

Embrace your healthy Journey to Motherhood
BONUS
I am confident in my ability to handle labor with ease."
Nuturing your inner strength today

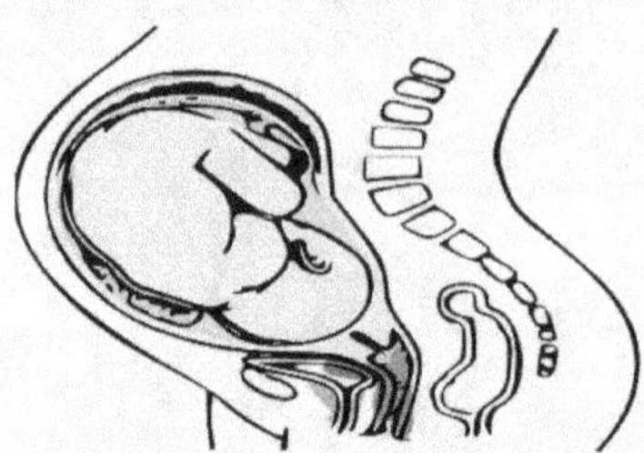

Embrace your healthy Journey to Motherhood
"Each wave of contraction brings me closer to my baby."
Nuturing your inner strength today
BONUS

Embrace your healthy Journey to Motherhood

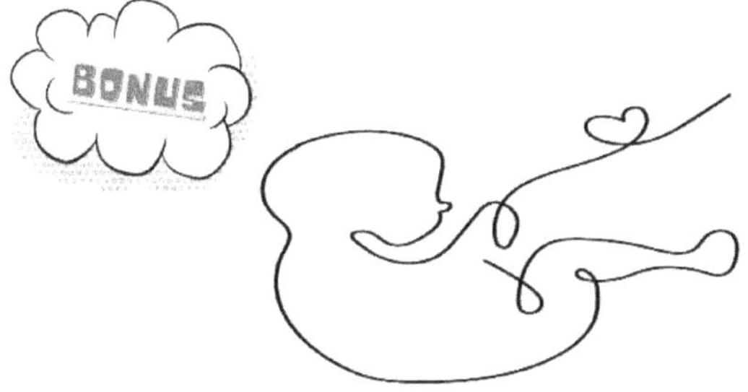

"I celebrate my strength and the miracle of life."

Nuturing your inner strength today

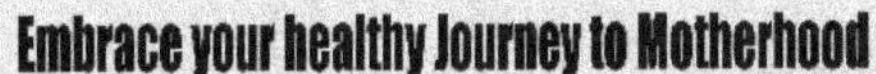

Embrace your healthy Journey to Motherhood

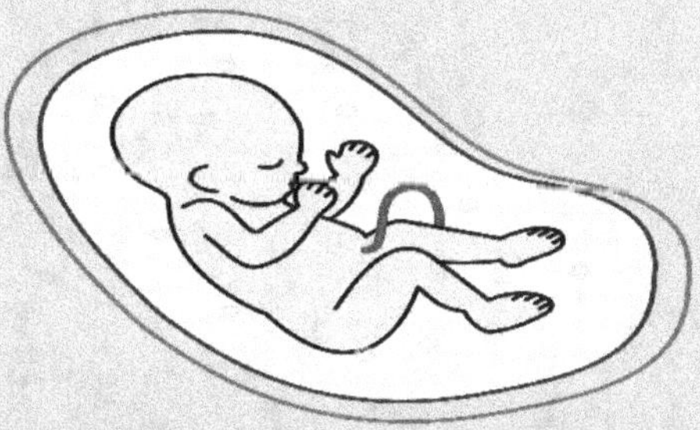

"My baby feels my love and calmness during this journey."

Nuturing your inner strength today

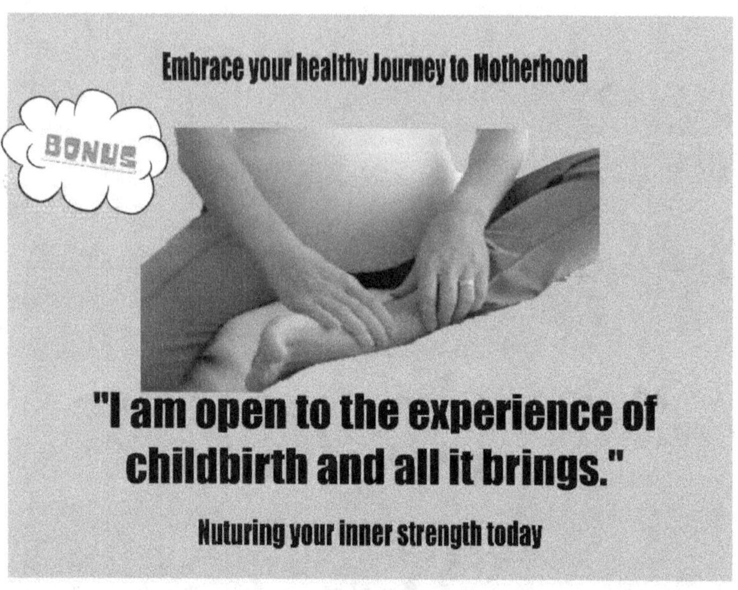
Embrace your healthy Journey to Motherhood
BONUS
"I am open to the experience of childbirth and all it brings."
Nuturing your inner strength today

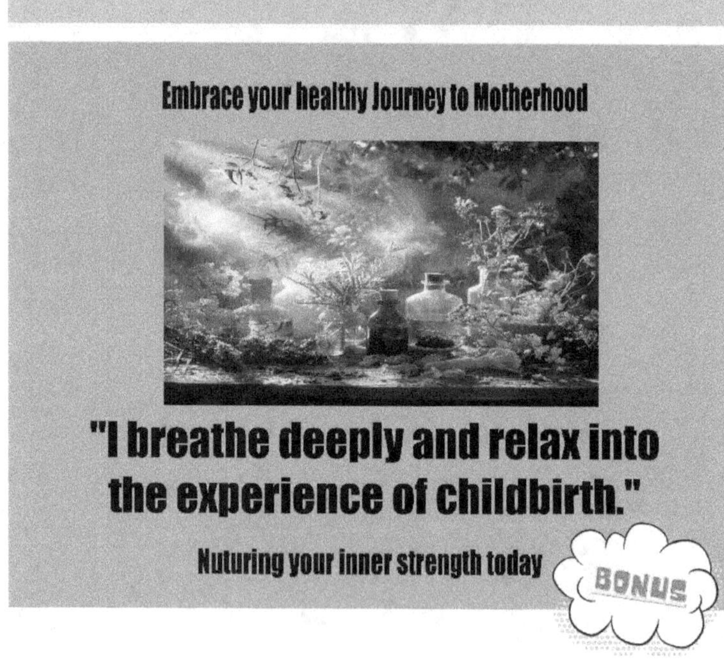
Embrace your healthy Journey to Motherhood
"I breathe deeply and relax into the experience of childbirth."
Nuturing your inner strength today
BONUS

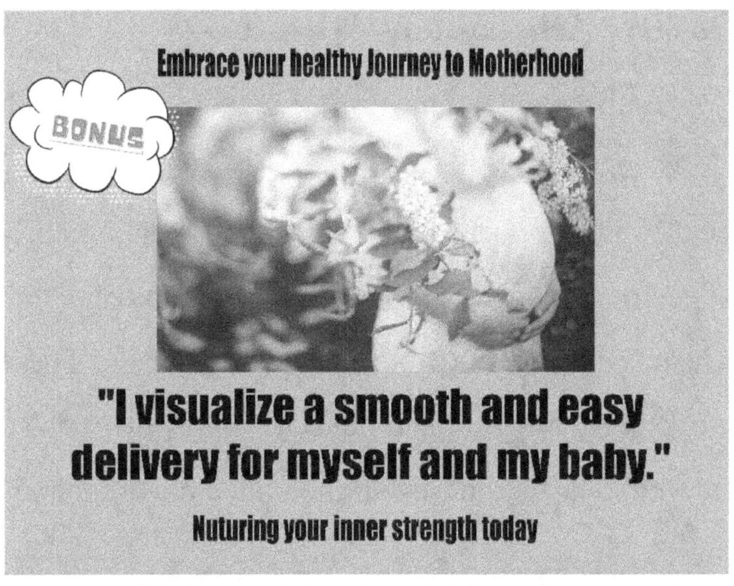
Embrace your healthy Journey to Motherhood
BONUS
"I visualize a smooth and easy delivery for myself and my baby."
Nuturing your inner strength today

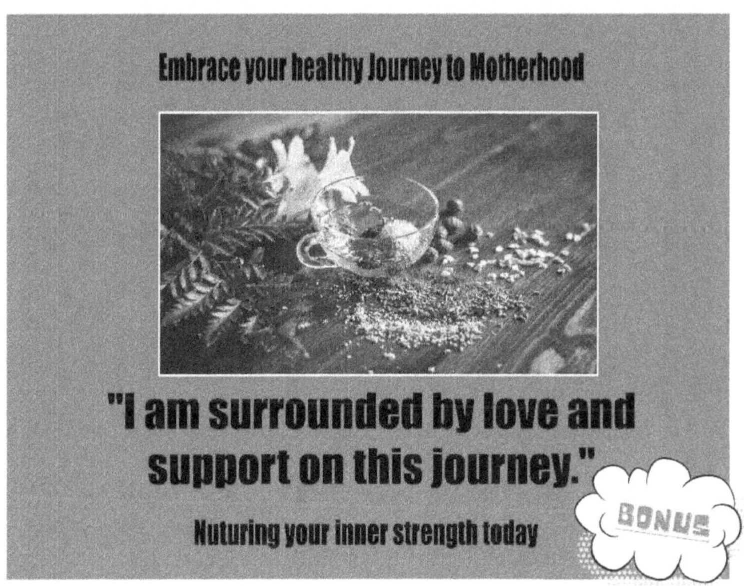
Embrace your healthy Journey to Motherhood
"I am surrounded by love and support on this journey."
Nuturing your inner strength today
BONUS

Positive Affirmations Worksheets

I recognize that the journey of pregnancy is as much about emotional well-being as it is about physical health. To support expectant mothers in cultivating a positive mindset, I have included colorful and illustrative positive affirmation worksheets. These worksheets are designed not only to inspire but also to empower you throughout your pregnancy journey.

What Are Positive Affirmation Worksheets?

Positive affirmation worksheets are interactive tools that help you engage with uplifting statements aimed at promoting self-confidence, reducing anxiety, and fostering a sense of calm. Each worksheet includes colorful illustrations and prompts that encourage you to reflect on your thoughts and feelings, making the practice of affirmations both enjoyable and impactful.

Importance of Using Affirmation Worksheets

1.Boosts Confidence: Regularly engaging with positive affirmations can help reinforce your belief in your abilities as a mother, especially during labor and delivery.

2.Reduces Anxiety: Focusing on positive thoughts can counteract feelings of fear or uncertainty, promoting emotional stability during pregnancy.

3.Encourages Mindfulness: Taking time to reflect on affirmations promotes mindfulness, helping you stay present and connected with your body and baby.

4.Fosters Creativity: The inclusion of coloring elements allows for creative expression, which can be therapeutic and relaxing.

How to Use the Positive Affirmation Worksheets

1.Set Aside Time: Dedicate a few quiet moments each day to engage with the worksheets. This could be in the morning to set positive intentions for the day or in the evening as a way to reflect on your experiences.

2.Choose Your Affirmations: Start by reading through the provided affirmations. Choose a few that resonate with you or inspire you. Feel free to modify them or create your own based on your personal experiences and feelings.

4.Daily Affirmation Tracker: Use the tracker section to write down your chosen affirmation for the day. At the end of the day, jot down how you felt when focusing on that affirmation—this helps reinforce positive thinking patterns.

5.Share Your Experience: If comfortable, share your completed worksheets with friends or family members who are also expecting. Discussing your affirmations can foster support and encouragement among peers.

6.Display Your Favorites: Select a few affirmations that resonate deeply with you and display them in visible areas of your home—on mirrors, bulletin boards, or even in your birthing space—to create an uplifting environment.

The positive affirmation worksheets included in "Herbal Recipes for Pregnancy" are more than just colorful pages; they are powerful tools designed to enhance your emotional well-being during pregnancy. By incorporating these worksheets into your daily routine, you can cultivate a mindset filled with positivity, confidence, and love as you prepare for motherhood.

WORSHEET

Complete the Sentences About You

1.   I am open to the experience ....

____

____

2.   My baby feels my love and ....

____

____

3.   I trust my body to know ....

____

____

4.   I celebrate my strength ....

____

____

I visualize a smooth and easy ....

---

5. **I am confident in my ability....**

---

6. **Each wave of contraction....**

---

7. **I am surrounded by love ....**

---

8. **I breathe deeply and relax ....**

9.   I am strong and capable ....

10.   I embrace each moment of labor....

11.   With every breath, I release....

12.   I trust the process and ....

13.   I am empowered by the strength....

____

____

14.   Every day, I grow stronger and....

____

____

15.   I welcome this experience....

____

____

16.   My body is perfectly designed....

____

____

17. I let go of fear and embrace ....

____

____

18. I am in tune with my body....

____

____

19. I am open to the experience ....

____

____

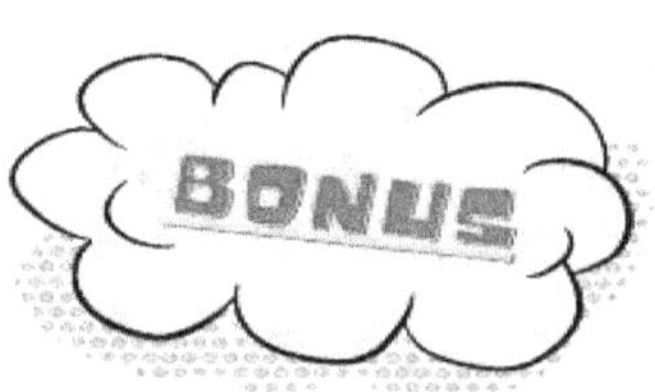

Other Positive Affirmatives

"My body is perfectly designed for this beautiful process."

"I embrace each moment of labor with courage and grace."

Every day, I grow stronger and more prepared for motherhood."

"I am in tune with my body and trust its wisdom."

"With every breath, I release tension and welcome calm."

 "I let go of fear and embrace the joy of bringing new life."

"I trust the process and remain focused on my goal."

"I am empowered by the strength of women before me."

"I welcome this experience with an open heart and mind."

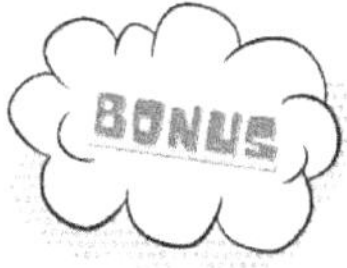

CONCLUSION

Embracing Natural Remedies in Your Pregnancy Journey

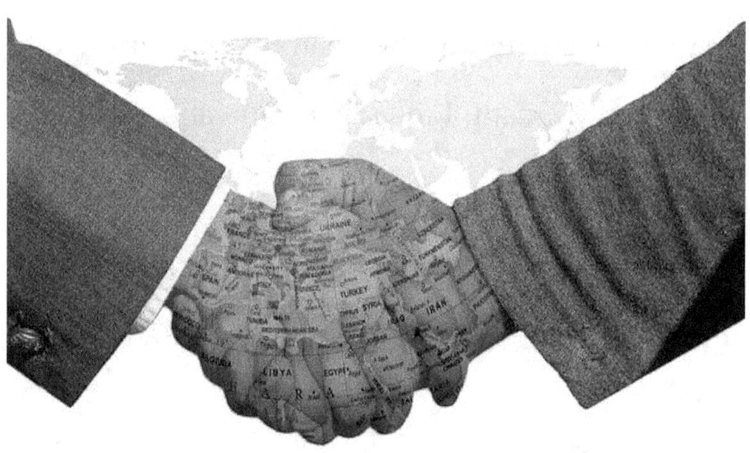

The journey through pregnancy is a transformative experience that brings about numerous physical and emotional changes. As expectant mothers navigate this path, embracing natural remedies can provide a holistic approach to wellness. Herbal remedies, when used thoughtfully and safely, can offer relief from common discomforts such as nausea, fatigue, and anxiety, while also supporting overall health.

Natural remedies allow mothers to connect with their bodies and the healing properties of plants. By incorporating safe herbs into their routines—such as ginger for nausea, chamomile for relaxation, and raspberry leaf for uterine support—expectant mothers can create a nurturing environment for themselves and their growing babies.

However, it is crucial to approach herbal remedies with caution. Consulting healthcare providers before using any herbal products ensures that mothers are informed about safety, potential interactions with medications, and appropriate dosages. This careful consideration helps maximize the benefits of herbal remedies while minimizing risks.

Final Thoughts on Herbal Wellness

Herbal wellness is not just about treating ailments; it's about fostering a deeper understanding of one's body and the natural world. Creating personalized herbal remedies allows individuals to tailor their health approaches to their specific needs. Whether through teas, tinctures, or topical applications, the process of making herbal remedies can be both empowering and educational.

As more people turn to herbal medicine for its perceived safety and efficacy, it's essential to prioritize quality and informed choices. Researching reputable sources for herbs, understanding the properties of different plants, and learning how to prepare them safely are vital steps in this journey.

In conclusion, embracing natural remedies during pregnancy can enhance wellbeing and provide comfort during this significant life transition. With proper guidance and knowledge, expectant mothers can confidently explore the world of herbal wellness, creating a supportive environment for themselves and their babies as they prepare for the joys of motherhood.

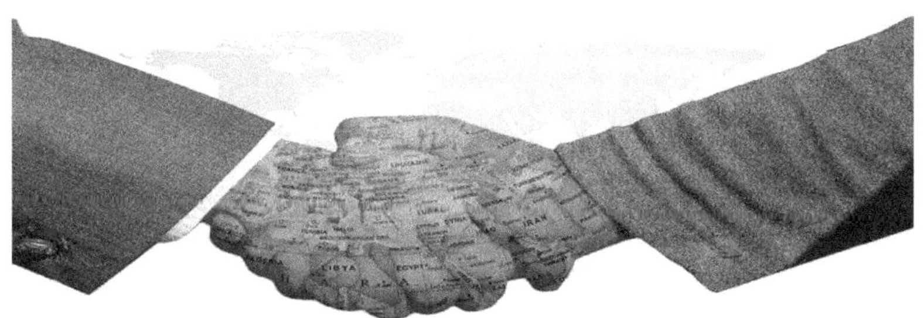